KT-471-170

The Midwife's Pocket Formulary

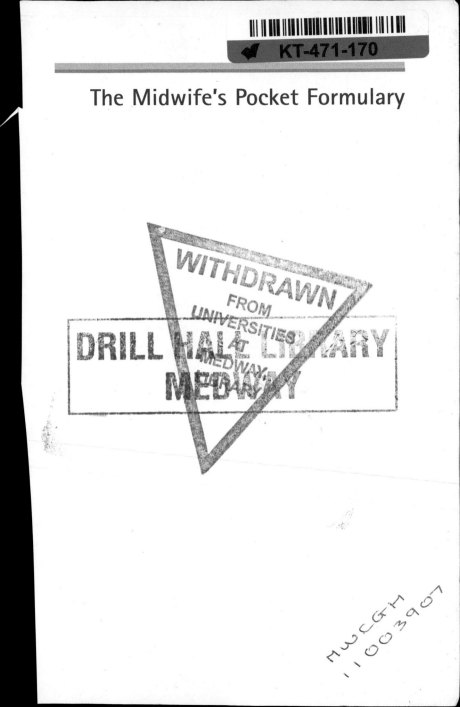

WITHDRAWN
FROM
UNIVERSITIES
AT
MEDWAY
LIBRARY

DRILL HALL LIBRARY
MEDWAY

MWCGH
1 003907

For Books for Midwives:

Commissioning Editor Mary Seager
Development Editor Catharine Steers
Project Controller Morven Dean
Designer George Ajayi

8017453

The Midwife's Pocket Formulary

Claire Banister RM

Midwife, Dorset County Hospital, Dorchester

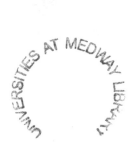

UNIVERSITIES AT MEDWAY LIBRARY

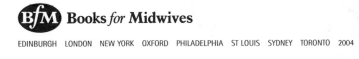

BfM **Books** *for* **Midwives**

EDINBURGH   LONDON   NEW YORK   OXFORD   PHILADELPHIA   ST LOUIS   SYDNEY   TORONTO   2004

BOOKS FOR MIDWIVES
An imprint of Elsevier Limited

© 2004, Elsevier Limited. All rights reserved.

No part of this publication may be reproduced, stored in a retrieval system, or transmitted in any form or by any means, electronic, mechanical, photocopying, recording or otherwise, without either the prior permission of the publishers or a licence permitting restricted copying in the United Kingdom issued by the Copyright Licensing Agency, 90 Tottenham Court Road, London W1T 4LP. Permissions may be sought directly from Elsevier's Health Sciences Rights Department in Philadelphia, USA: phone: (+1) 215 238 7869, fax: (+1) 215 238 2239, e-mail: healthpermissions@elsevier.com. You may also complete your request on-line via the Elsevier Science homepage (http://www.elsevier.com), by selecting 'Customer Support' and then 'Obtaining Permissions'.

First published 2004

ISBN 0750688033

British Library Cataloguing in Publication Data
A catalogue record for this book is available from the British Library

Library of Congress Cataloging in Publication Data
A catalog record for this book is available from the Library of Congress

Notice
Medical knowledge is constantly changing. Standard safety precautions must be followed, but as new research and clinical experience broaden our knowledge, changes in treatment and drug therapy may become necessary or appropriate. Readers are advised to check the most current product information provided by the manufacturer of each drug to be administered to verify the recommended dose, the method and duration of administration, and contraindications. It is the responsibility of the practitioner, relying on experience and knowledge of the patient, to determine dosages and the best treatment for each individual patient. Neither the publisher nor the editor assumes any liability for any injury and/or damage to persons or property arising from this publication.

The Publisher

Printed and bound in the United Kingdom

Transferred to Digital Print 2011

UNIVERSITIES AT MEDWAY
02 DEC 2011
DRILL HALL LIBRARY

The
publisher's
policy is to use
**paper manufactured
from sustainable forests**

Contents

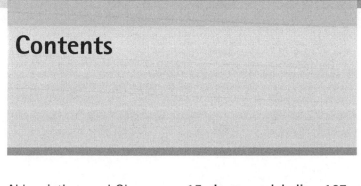

Abbreviations and Glossary of Terms

b.d.	bis die – twice a day
t.d.s.	ter die sumendus – three times a day
q.d.s.	quatre die sumendus – four times a day
nocte	at night
stat	immediately
p.r.n.	pro re nata – as the need arises
hrly	hourly
IM	intramuscular – of injections
IV	intravenous
IVI	intravenous infusion
p.o.	per os – by mouth
p.r.	per rectum – rectally
p.v.	per vaginam – vaginally
s.c.	subcutaneous – of injections
mg	milligrams
g	grams
kg	kilogram
ml	millilitre
l	litre
APTT	Activated Partial Prothrombin Time – used to monitor clotting when anticoagulant used is heparin
ARM	Artificial Rupture of Membranes
BNF	*British National Formulary*
CD	Controlled Drug
CNS	Central Nervous System
DCT	Direct Coombes Test

DVT   Deep Vein Thrombosis

eMC   *electronic Medicines Compendium*

GABA   Gamma-AminoButyric Acid – a deficiency of this inhibitory neurotransmitter may cause excessive responses to excitatory factors and may play a part in the initiation of abnormal discharge, and ultimately convulsions

GSL   General Sales List

HDN   Haemorrhagic Disease of the Newborn

INR   International Normalized Ratio – usually used to monitor prothrombin time when anticoagulant used is warfarin

IUCD   Intrauterine Contraceptive Device

IUD   Intrauterine Death

LMWH   Low Molecular Weight Heparin

LSCS   Lower-Segment Caesarean Section

MAOI   Monoamine Oxidase Inhibitor – a drug that prevents the breakdown of serotonin, leading to an increase in mental and physical activity

MRP   Manual Removal of Placenta

MRSA   Methicillin-Resistant *Staphylococcus Aureus*

NSAID   Non-Steroidal Anti-Inflammatory Drug – a drug that inhibits the production of prostaglandins and which has antipyretic, anti-inflammatory and analgesic properties

OCP   Oral Contraceptive Pill

P   Pharmacy-Only Medicine

PDA   Patent Ductus Arteriosus

POM   Prescription-Only Medicine

SLE   Systemic Lupus Erythematosus

SRM   Spontaneous Rupture of Membranes

SSRI   Selective Serotonin Reuptake Inhibitor – these drugs inhibit the reuptake of serotonin at nerve terminals, leading to inhibition of excitatory impulses and subsequent overload, and are used in conditions such as depression, anxiety and panic disorders

TCA   Tricyclic Antidepressants – complex action but thought to inhibit the uptake and reuptake of serotonin and noradrenaline (norepinephrine)

UFH   Unfractionated Heparin

URTI   Upper Respiratory Tract Infection

UTI   Urinary Tract Infection

Anticholinergic – a drug that inhibits the effects of acetylcholine, a chemical transmitter released by some nerve endings at the synapse between one neuron and another, or the nerve endings and the effector organ. It supplies the lower motor neurons and parasympathetic nerves. Anticholinergic drugs relax smooth muscle, are antispasmodics, and inhibit secretory responses and vomiting

Antimuscarinic – a synthetic anticholinergic drug; the opposite of a muscarinic drug

Extrapyramidal – affecting the nerve tracts outside the pyramidal (spinal) tract

Muscarinic – causes sympathetic symptoms, i.e. the actions of acetylcholine on the nerve endings and the sympathetic nerves; e.g. increases salivation, bronchial secretions, gastrointestinal activity

Myasthenia gravis – an extreme form of muscle weakness, thought to be related to the rapid destruction of acetylcholine at neurotransmitter junctions

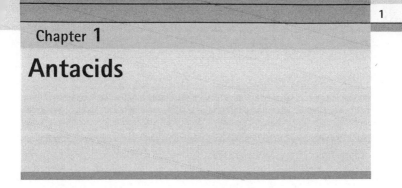

Chapter 1

Antacids

These drugs/preparations are used to reduce gastric acidity and give relief from heartburn when changes in diet and posture have no effect. They may also be used as prophylaxis prior to the induction of anaesthesia where there is a risk of Mendelsson's syndrome, i.e. prior to either elective or emergency caesarean section.

Antacids should not be taken at the same time as other medication as they impair absorption.

H_2 antagonists act upon histamine receptors and can intensify or aggravate an asthmatic response, and should be used with caution in hepatic and or renal impairment.

The student should be aware of:

- The effect of progesterone on the mother
- Local protocols for management of high-risk clients during labour
- The procedure of applying 'cricoid pressure' during induction of anaesthesia
- Updated resuscitation techniques
- The effects of narcotic analgesia on gastric emptying.

References

Briggs GG, Freeman RK, Yaffe SJ. Drugs in pregnancy and lactation: a reference guide to fetal and neonatal risk, 3rd edn. Baltimore: Williams and Wilkins, 1990

British Medical Association and Royal Pharmaceutical Society of Great Britain. British national formulary, March 2002 Number 43. Bath: Bath Press, 2002

Enkin M, Kierse MJNC, Neilson J et al. (eds) A guide to effective care in pregnancy and childbirth, 3rd edn. Oxford: Oxford University Press, 2000; 99, 260–263, 265

Hale T. Medications and mothers' milk, 9th edn. USA: Pharmasoft Publishing, 2000

Henney CR, Dow RJ, MacConnachie AM. Drugs in nursing practice: A–Z guide. Edinburgh: Churchill Livingstone, 1995

Hopkins SJ. Drugs and pharmacology for nurses, 13th edn. Edinburgh: Churchill Livingstone, 1999

SPC from the eMC Zantac® 150 mg, GlaxoWellcome, updated on the eMC 15/08/01

SPC from the eMC Tagamet® 800 mg, 400 mg, effervescent tablets 400 mg, syrup, injection, SmithKline Beecham, updated on the eMC 21/08/01

SPC from the eMC Liquid Gaviscon®; Liquid Gaviscon® – peppermint flavour, Britannia Pharmaceuticals Ltd, updated on the eMC 28/08/01

Stockley IH (ed) Drug interactions, 5th edn. London: Pharmaceutical Press 1999

Further Reading

Enkin M, Kierse MJNC, Neilson J et al. (eds) A guide to effective care in pregnancy and childbirth, 3rd edn. Oxford: Oxford University Press, 2000; 99, 260–263, 265

Lewis G, Drife J. Why mothers die 1997–1999. The confidential enquiries into maternal deaths in the United Kingdom. London: RCOG Press, 2001

Vamer RG. Mechanisms of regurgitation and its prevention with cricoid pressure. International Journal of Obstetrical Anaesthesia 1993; 2:207–215

BP	RANITIDINE
Proprietary	Zantac® (Glaxo Wellcome), contains sodium
Group	antacid, H_2 antagonist
Uses/indications	reduces gastric acidity in high-risk labours, prior to caesarean section or any other surgical procedure
Type of drug	POM
Presentation	tablets (also dispersible or effervescent), syrup, injection
Dosage	150 mg at onset of labour, repeat 6 hrly or see protocols, IM or slow IV 50 mg 45–60 minutes prior to the induction of analgesia, IV injection 20 mL over 2 minutes
Route of admin	oral, IM, IV injection
Contraindications	as for cimetidine, hypersensitivity
Side effects	as for cimetidine, rarely tachycardia, and with long-term use agitation and visual disturbances
Interactions	as for cimetidine, but effects less likely
Pharmacodynamic properties	as for cimetidine, relatively long acting. 150 mg suppresses gastric acidity for 12 hrs
Fetal risk	crosses the placenta and should only be used in the long term if essential, for prophylaxis in labour or LSCS. No adverse effect has been reported on labour, delivery or neonatal period
Breastfeeding	excreted in significant amounts but not known to be harmful

BP	CIMETIDINE
Proprietary	Dyspamet® (Gold Shield), Tagamet® (SmithKline Beecham), cimetidine (non-proprietary)
Group	antacid, H_2 receptor antagonist
Uses/indications	to reduce gastric acidity, intrapartum or prior to caesarean section
Type of drug	POM (GSL – Tagamet® –100 mg)
Presentation	tablets – light green, also chewable and effervescent, IM injection, syrup
Dosage	oral – 400 mg at start of labour repeated 4 hrly (max 2.4 g/day) IM – 200 mg 4–6 hrly (max dosage 2.4 g daily), IV – slow injection 200 mg over at least 5 minutes 4–6 hrly, IVI – 50–100 mg/h over 24 hrs
Route of admin	oral, IM, rarely IV slow injection or IVI
Contraindications	hypersensitivity to cimetidine, avoid in clients stabilized on phenytoin and warfarin
Side effects	rare but include dizziness, rash, in high doses reversible confusional states, headache
Interactions	*analgesics* – inhibits the metabolism of opioid analgesics and increases their plasma concentration *antibiotics* – inhibits the metabolism of metronidazole and erythromycin *anticoagulants* – inhibits the metabolism of warfarin, and enhances its effects *antiepileptics* – inhibits the metabolism of phenytoin, sodium valproate and carbamazepine *antihypertensives* – inhibits the metabolism of labetalol

table continues

Pharmacodynamic properties	H_2 receptor antagonist which rapidly inhibits both basal and stimulated gastric secretion of acid. It also reduces pepsin output
Fetal risk	no evidence to suggest cimetidine is hazardous but it should be avoided unless necessary
Breastfeeding	excreted in breast milk but not known to be harmful

BP	ALGINIC ACID
Proprietary	Gaviscon® (Britannia Pharmaceuticals Ltd)
Group	Antacid – alginate
Uses/indications	dyspepsia, cardiac reflux (heartburn)
Type of drug	GSL
Presentation	tablets, oral suspension – peppermint, lemon or aniseed
Dosage	tablets 1–2 as required, or 10–20 mL as required
Route of admin	oral
Contraindications	no data available
Side effects	no data available, but caution in a sodium-restricted diet
Interactions	impaired absorption of oral iron
Pharmacodynamic properties	Alginic acid reacts with the gastric acid to form a pH neutral gel raft over the stomach contents and is effective for up to 4 hrs
Fetal risk	nil known
Breastfeeding	not secreted in breast milk

Chapter 2

Anaesthesia

These drugs depress part of the central nervous system, causing the loss of sensation in a part of or in the whole of the body.

There are two main groups, inhalational and intravenous.

These drugs are the speciality of an anaesthetist, although midwives do use certain ones, e.g. nitrous oxide via Entonox, or local agents such as lignocaine for perineal infiltration and bupivacaine for epidural top-ups. This chapter explores those anaesthetics used by midwives and not those administered by anaesthetists alone.

It is also of note that in the 1997–99 Confidential Enquiries into Maternal Deaths in the UK (Lewis and Drife 2001) anaesthesia was directly responsible for three deaths (3%), although anaesthesia contributed to 21 (a considerable number), several of which were due to lack of careful monitoring.

Midwives need to be aware of the action of anaesthetics and units need to provide recovery areas for CS patients and high-risk clients.

The student should be aware of:

- The difference between analgesia and anaesthesia
- The difference between local, regional and general anaesthesia
- The physiology and pathophysiology of the perception of pain
- The physiological principles underpinning epidural anaesthesia

- Problems that occur with obstetrical anaesthesia, i.e. the effects of progesterone on the mother, the presence of two patients rather than one, the pressure of the gravid uterus
- Updated resuscitation techniques
- How to apply cricoid pressure if requested to in an emergency.

References

Bevis R. Obstetric anaesthesia and operations. In: Bennett VR, Brown LK, eds. Myles textbook for midwives, 13th edn. Edinburgh: Churchill Livingstone, 1999; Chapter 28, pp 539–552

Briggs GG, Freeman RK, Yaffe SJ. Drugs in pregnancy and lactation : a reference guide to fetal and neonatal risk, 3rd edn. Baltimore: Williams & Wilkins, 1990

British Medical Association and the Royal Pharmaceutical Society of Great Britain. British national formulary. Number 43, March 2002. Bath: Bath Press, 2002

Hale T. Medications and mothers' milk, 9th edn. USA: Pharmasoft Publications, 2000

Hopkins SJ. Drugs and pharmacology for nurses, 13th edn. Edinburgh: Churchill Livingstone, 1999

Lewis G, Drife J. Why mothers die 1997–1999. The confidential enquiries into maternal deaths in the UK. London: RCOG Press, 2001

Stockley IH (ed) Drug interactions, 5th edn. London: Pharmaceutical Press, 1999

SPC from the eMC, Marcain® Heavy, AstraZeneca, updated on the eMC 17/08/01

SPC from the eMC, Xylocaine™ Antiseptic Gel 2%, Xylocaine™ Accordion Antiseptic Gel 2%, AstraZeneca, 14/02/02

SPC from the eMC, Marcain® Polyamp Steripack 0.5%, AstraZeneca, updated on the eMC

SPC from the eMC, Emla® Cream AstraZeneca updated on the eMC 11/02/02

SPC from BOC gases, Entonox™, BOC Gases Ltd, 07/04/00

Further Reading and Research

Bevis R. Anaesthesia in midwifery. London: Baillière Tindall, 1984

Dennis AR, Leeson-Payne CG, Langham BT, Aitkenhead AR. Local anaesthesia for cannulation: Has practice changed? Anaesthesia 1995;50:400–402

Mahajan J, Mahajan RP, Singh MM et al. Anaesthetic technique for elective caesarean section and neurobehavioural status of the newborn. International Journal of Obstetric Anaesthesia 1993;2:89–93

Sepkoski CM, Lester BM, Ostheimer GW, Brazleton TB. The effects of maternal epidural anaesthesia on neonatal behaviour during the first month. Developmental Medicine and Child Neurology 1992;34:1072–1080

Vamer RG. Mechanisms of regurgitation and its prevention with cricoid pressure. International Journal of Obstetric Anaesthesia 1993;2:207–215

BP	NITROUS OXIDE
Proprietary	Entonox™ (BOC Gases)
Group	anaesthetic, inhalational
Uses/indications	analgesia during labour
Type of drug	POM, standing orders
Presentation	colourless gas with slightly sweet odour in cylinders – blue with blue and white quarters at the valve end and labelled Entonox™
Dosage	50% nitrous oxide: 50% oxygen, self-administered via mask or Entonox™ equipment
Route of admin	inhalational
Contraindications	pneumothorax, facial or jaw injuries, diving accidents, overt drunkenness
Side effects	drowsiness, nausea, vomiting
Interactions	none specific, but BNF (2001) indicates that it may be appropriate to consider that it enhances the effect of other anaesthetics or analgesics, and is similar in action to a general anaesthetic. Relevant interactions to obstetrics are that: *anxiolytics and hypnotics* – enhances the sedative effect *Methyldopa* – increases the hypotensive effect
Fetal risk	can depress neonatal respiration (BNF 2001). It is also of note that it may increase the risk of spontaneous abortion and low birthweight in female workers where levels of exposure are raised, i.e. operating theatres, labour wards
Breastfeeding	No data available on controlled studies during breastfeeding

BP	LIGNOCAINE HYDROCHLORIDE
Proprietary	Xylocaine™ (AstraZeneca)
Group	local anaesthetic
Uses/indications	perineal infiltration – prior to episiotomy or suturing, or for nerve blocks
Type of drug	POM, standing orders
Presentation	glass or polypropylene ampoules 2, 5, 10 or 20 mL, with strength, 1% or 2%, indicated on the ampoule
Dosage	as per unit protocol, lowest concentration and smallest dose producing the required effect
Route of admin	injection
Contraindications	hypersensitivity and profound hypovolaemia
Side effects	hypotension, bradycardia, hypersensitivity can lead to anaphylaxis, although this is rare, also inadvertent IV injection can lead to central nervous system excitatory response and then drowsiness, convulsions and respiratory arrest
Interactions	(less likely when used topically) *anaesthetics* – action of suxamethonium is prolonged, bupivacaine increases the risk of myocardial depression *antacids* – cimetidine increases the plasma concentration absorption of lignocaine and can increase the risk of toxicity *antipsychotics* – increased risk of toxicity with myelosuppressive drugs *β blockers* – increased risk of myocardial depression with propranolol

table continues

Pharmacodynamic properties	stabilizes the neuronal membrane and prevents the initiation and conduction of nerve impulses, causing profound anaesthesia of the membranes and lubrication that reduces friction. Effective in 5 minutes and lasts for 20–30 minutes
Fetal risk	after large doses neonatal respiratory depression, hypertonia, bradycardia after paracervical block, or accidental direct injection during infiltration of the perineum prior to episiotomy
Breastfeeding	No data available on controlled studies during breastfeeding

BP	BUPIVACAINE HYDROCHLORIDE
Proprietary	Marcain® (AstraZeneca) Marcain Heavy® (AstraZeneca)
Group	local anaesthetic
Uses/indications	epidural anaesthesia, spinal anaesthesia
Type of drug	POM
Presentation	polypropylene ampoules (Steripacks) of differing percentages
Dosage	as prescribed by the anaesthetist
Route of admin	intrathecal injection
Contraindications	hypovolaemia, hypotension, pyrexia in labour, pyogenic infection of the skin at or adjacent to the lumbar site, coagulation disorders or ongoing coagulation treatment, known hypersensitivity to local anaesthetics such as lignocaine, meningitis, hypovolaemic shock, intracranial haemorrhage, cardiogenic shock, low levels of platelets
Side effects	anaphylaxis, maternal hypotension, bradycardia – preloading with crystalloids required – persistent or profound symptoms can be reversed with ephedrine 10–15 mg IV, myocardial depression and seizures if given IV, may cause maternal pyrexia and some diminishing of uterine contractions, post lumbar headache. A high block causes respiratory embarrassment, arrest and paralysis. Neurological problems include paraesthesia, motor weakness and loss of sphincter control

table continues

	accidental IV injection – causes numbness of the tongue, tinnitus, light-headedness, dizziness and tremors, followed by drowsiness, convulsions and cardiac disorders, and requires the attendance of skilled anaesthetic help
Interactions	*antiarrythmics* – increased myocardial depression
Pharmacodynamic properties	Marcain Heavy® – local anaesthetic of the amide type which causes moderate relaxation of lower extremities and a motor blockade of abdominal muscles bupivacaine – as above, but analgesia without the motor blockade
Fetal risk	reportedly bradycardia, respiratory depression, fetal hypothermia. Toxicity in animal studies indicates avoidance in early pregnancy, but manufacturers suggest there is no evidence of untoward effects
Breastfeeding	excreted in small amounts but no risk from therapeutic doses

BP	LIGNOCAINE HYDROCHLORIDE 2.5%: PRILOCAINE 2.5%
Proprietary	EMLA 5% CREAM™ (AstraZeneca)
Group	anaesthetic – local
Uses/indications	anaesthesia prior to venepuncture, surface analgesia
Type of drug	POM
Presentation	white soft cream
Dosage	thick layer 1–5 hours prior to procedure under occlusive dressing
Route of admin	topical
Contraindications	dermatitis at site, mucous membrane, wounds or hypersensitivity to active constituents
Side effects	transient paleness, redness and oedema have been reported
Interactions	as for lignocaine, but unlikely
Pharmacodynamic properties	provides dermal analgesia, depending on application time and dose, by causing transient local vasoconstriction or vasodilation at the treated area
Fetal risk	crosses the placental barrier, but no ill effects have been reported
Breastfeeding	excreted in breast milk in small amounts but considered safe

BP	LIGNOCAINE HYDROCHLORIDE
Proprietary	Xylocaine antiseptic gel (AstraZeneca)
Group	anaesthetic – local
Uses/indications	anaesthesia of the urethra prior to catheterization, or topical application to mucous membranes, i.e. the perineum
Type of drug	POM
Presentation	ampoules of gel or in accordion gel pack
Dosage	5–10 ml intraurethrally to fill urethra
Route of admin	topical/intraurethral
Contraindications	hypersensitivity to lignocaine. Trauma to the urethra can cause increased systemic absorption
Side effects	as for lignocaine but less, as topically applied
Interactions	as for lignocaine, but unlikely
Pharmacodynamic properties	stabilizes the neuronal membrane and prevents the initiation and conduction of nerve impulses, causing profound anaesthesia of the membranes and lubrication that reduces friction. Effective in 5 minutes and lasts for 20–30 minutes
Fetal risk	no evidence of harm but avoid in early pregnancy
Breastfeeding	no evidence of risk

Chapter 3

Analgesics

These preparations are used to relieve pain without causing unconsciousness or lack of all nervous sensation in a particular area. It is important to become familiar with pain theories and to use the body's natural analgesics to their optimum effect, as well as using chemical preparations.

The student should be aware of:

- Pain theories, especially the 'gate theory' of Melzack and Wall (1964)
- The difference between anaesthesia and analgesia
- The accumulative effect of many analgesics, which can lead to intentional or accidental overdose
- The different combinations of separate analgesic compounds
- The possibility of addiction to analgesics
- Neonatal sequelae to maternal analgesia
- The appropriateness of the analgesic compound to the complaint.

References

Bevis R. Pain relief and comfort in labour. In: Bennett VR, Brown LK, eds. Myles textbook for midwives, 13th edn. Edinburgh: Churchill Livingstone, 1999; 429–446

Briggs GG, Freeman RK, Yaffe SJ. Drugs in pregnancy and lactation : a reference guide to fetal and neonatal risk, 3rd edn. Baltimore: Williams & Wilkins,1990

British Medical Association and the Royal Pharmaceutical Society of Great Britain. British national formulary. Number 43, March 2002. Bath: Bath Press, 2002

Hale T. Medications and mothers' milk, 9th edn. USA: Pharmasoft Publications, 2000

Hopkins SJ. Drugs and pharmacology for nurses, 3th edn. Edinburgh: Churchill Livingstone, 1999

Little BB. Medication in pregnancy. In: James DK, Steer PJ, Weiner CP, Gonik B (eds) High risk pregnancy: management options, 2nd edn. London: WB Saunders, 1999; 617–638

Niven C. Coping with labour pain: the midwife's role. In: Robinson S, Thompson AM, eds. Midwives, research and childbirth. Vol 3. London: Chapman & Hall, 1994; 91–119

PIL from the eMC, Buscopan® tablets, Boehringer Ingelheim Ltd, last revised January 1999

SPC from the eMC, Soluble Aspirin BP Tablets 300 mg, Boots Company PLC, updated on eMC 18/12/01

SPC from the eMC, Paracetamol Caplets 500 mg, Boots Company PLC, updated on eMC 15/11/01

SPC from the eMC, Tylex® Effervescent, Schwartz Pharma Ltd, updated on the eMC 3/08/01

SPC from the eMC, Co-Codamol BP effervescent tablets, Lagap Pharmaceuticals Ltd, revision of the text, September 1997

SPC from the eMC, Distalgesic®, Dista Products Ltd, updated on the eMC 13/08/01

SPC from the eMC, Solpadol® Capsules, Solpadol® effervescent tablets, Solpadol® caplets, Sanofi Synthelabo, updated on the eMC 22/08/01

SPC from the eMC, Diclofenac Sodium BP tablets 50 mg, Pharmacia, updated on the eMC 25/08/01

SPC from the eMC, Ponstan™ Capsules 250 mg, Chemidex Pharma Ltd, updated on the eMC 2/04/02

SPC from the eMC, Morphine Sulphate Injection BP 100 mg in 1 mL, 15 mg in 1 mL, 30 mg in 1 mL, Celltech Pharmaceuticals Ltd, updated on the eMC 23/08/01

SPC from the eMC, Sublimaze®, Janssen-Cilag Ltd, updated on the eMC 17/08/01

SPC from the eMC, Nurofen®, Crookes Healthcare Ltd, updated on the eMC 26/07/01

SPC from the eMC, Paramol®, SSL International, updated on the
   eMC 3/07/01
SPC from the eMC, Paramol® (new capsule shape), SSL
   International, updated on the eMC 17/04/02
Stockley IH (ed). Drug interactions, 5th edn. London:
   Pharmaceutical Press, 1999

Further Reading

Yerby M. Managing pain in labour Pt 2: Non-pharmacological pain
   relief. Modern Midwife 1996; 6:16–18
Yerby M. Managing pain in labour Pt 3: Pharmacological methods
   of pain relief. Modern Midwife 1996; 6:22–25

BP	CO-CODAPRIN
Proprietary	Co-codaprin (non-proprietary; see BNF for details)
Group	analgesic, aspirin compound (aspirin 400 mg + codeine phosphate 8 mg
Uses/indications	mild to moderate pain
Type of drug	POM
Presentation	tablets (white)
Dosage	1–2 tablets 4–6-hrly (max. 8 daily)
Route of admin	oral
Contraindications	as for codeine and aspirin
Side effects	as for codeine and aspirin
Interactions	as for codeine and aspirin
Fetal risk	as for codeine and aspirin
Breastfeeding	should be avoided in view of aspirin content, although there are no controlled studies available for breastfeeding women

BP	CO–DYDRAMOL (PARACETAMOL 500 MG + DIHYDROCODEINE 10 MG)
Proprietary	Paramol® (SSL International – paracetamol 521 mg + dihydrocodeine 7.46 mg)
Group	analgesic, paracetamol and opioid compound
Uses/indications	mild to moderate pain
Type of drug	POM, GSL
Presentation	tablets (white)
Dosage	1–2 tablets 4–6-hrly (max. 8 daily)
Route of admin	oral
Contraindications	as for paracetamol and dihydrocodeine
Side effects	as for paracetamol and dihydrocodeine
Interactions	as for paracetamol and dihydrocodeine
Fetal risk	as for dihydrocodeine
Breastfeeding	no controlled study data available for breastfeeding and the risk of untoward effects in a breastfed infant is a possibility. The compound is considered safe, as it is taken by a large number of women with no observed increase in adverse effects in infants

BP	CO-PROXAMOL (PARACETAMOL 325 MG + DEXTROPROPOXYPHENE 32.5 MG)
Proprietary	Distalgesic® (Dista Products Ltd)
Group	analgesic, compound of paracetamol and opioid salt
Uses/indications	mild to moderate pain
Type of drug	POM (CD Schedule 5), GSL
Presentation	tablets (white marked DG)
Dosage	1–2 tablets 4–6–hrly (max. 8 daily)
Route of admin	oral
Contraindications	alcohol abuse, hypersensitivity to either of the constituents, addictive or suicidal clients, hepatic or renal impairment, concomitant paracetamol usage
Side effects	dizziness, sedation, nausea, vomiting, constipation, abdominal pain, headache. NB: *overdose* is complicated by respiratory depression, heart failure and by hepatic failure, and *can cause death in 15 minutes*
Interactions	CNS depressant effect of the opioid constituent enhances the effect of CNS depressants, including alcohol *anticoagulant* – effect of warfarin possibly enhanced *anticonvulsants* – altered metabolism – see above *antidepressants* – altered metabolism – see above

table continues

Pharmacodynamic properties	a compound analgesic with a non-narcotic (paracetamol) for relief of pain in musculoskeletal conditions and a narcotic (dextropropoxyphene) for relief of visceral pain
Fetal risk	not established as safe in pregnancy, withdrawal reported in neonates. Potential benefits should outweigh the possible hazards
Breastfeeding	amount secreted too small to be harmful

BP	CO-CODAMOL (PARACETAMOL 500 MG + CODEINE 8 MG)
Proprietary	Solpadol® (Sanofi Synthelabo), Tylex™ (Schwartz Pharma Ltd) (paracetamol 500 mg + codeine 30 mg)
Group	analgesic, paracetamol and opioid compound
Uses/indications	mild to moderate pain
Type of drug	POM, GSL
Presentation	tablets, capsules, dispersible tablets
Dosage	1–2 tablets or capsules 4-hrly, max. 8 daily
Route of admin	oral
Contraindications	as for paracetamol and codeine
Side effects	as for paracetamol and codeine phosphate
Interactions	as for paracetamol and codeine phosphate
Fetal risk	as for codeine phosphate
Breastfeeding	no controlled study data available for breastfeeding and the risk of untoward effects in a breastfed infant is a possibility. The compound is considered safe, as it is taken by a large number of women with no observed increase in adverse effects in infants

BP	IBUPROFEN
Proprietary	Brufen® (Knoll), (GSL – Nurofen® Crookes Healthcare Ltd) ibuprofen (non-proprietary, see BNF for details)
Group	analgesic, non-opioid, NSAID
Uses/indications	mild to moderate pain, particularly perineal
Type of drug	POM, GSL
Presentation	tablets, syrup, granules
Dosage	1.2–1.8 g daily in 3–4 doses (after food)
Route of admin	oral
Contraindications	pregnancy, salicylate hypersensitivity, asthma
Side effects	gastrointestinal discomfort, diarrhoea, nausea, rash, headache, dizziness
Interactions	as for diclofenac and salicylic acid
Pharmacodynamic properties	analgesic, anti-inflammatory, antipyretic, this NSAID is thought to act by inhibiting prostaglandin synthesis
Fetal risk	as for salicylic acid, delayed onset and increased duration of labour
Breastfeeding	apparently safe

BP	MEFENAMIC ACID
Proprietary	Ponstan™ (Chemidex Pharma Ltd)
Group	analgesic, non-opioid, NSAID
Uses/indications	mild to moderate pain, postpartum pain, postoperative pain, anti-inflammatory
Type of drug	POM
Presentation	tablets, capsules
Dosage	500 mg t.d.s. after food
Route of admin	oral
Contraindications	hypersensitivity to mefenamic acid, irritable bowel syndrome, peptic/intestinal ulceration, renal or hepatic impairment, asthma or allergic reactions, i.e. rhinitis or urticaria or bronchospasm on administration of NSAIDs
Side effects	drowsiness, diarrhoea, nausea, rash, thrombocytopenia, haemolytic anaemia or purpuric rash. If these occur withdraw the drug. Hypersensitive reaction – bronchospasm, urticaria, nausea, vomiting abdominal pain, headache facial oedema, laryngeal oedema, dizziness, abnormal vision, palpitations
Interactions	as for diclofenac, but especially *anticoagulants* – increased effect *antihypertensives* – reduces the hypotensive effect OVERDOSE – can cause convulsions

table continues

Pharmacodynamic properties	a prostaglandin synthesis inhibiting NSAID with anti-inflammatory, antipyretic effects and analgesic properties
Fetal risk	safety is not established and possibly has same effects as salicylic acid
Breastfeeding	insufficient information to allow breastfeeding safely

BP	PARACETAMOL (ACETAMINOPHEN)
Proprietary	paracetamol (refer to BNF for manufacturers and advice on trade names)
Group	analgesic, non-opioid
Uses/indications	mild to moderate pain, headache, rheumatic pains, pyrexia
Type of drug	POM, GSL (sold to the public in packs of no more than 32; pharmacists may dispense up to 100)
Presentation	tablets, oral suspension, dispersible tablets, suppositories
Dosage	oral: 500 mg–1 g 4–6-hrly (max. 4 g daily) p.r. 0.5–1 g q.d.s.
Route of admin	oral, p.r.
Contraindications	hypersensitivity, hepatic and renal disease, alcohol dependence
Side effects	*rare,* blood disorders, rashes, overdose causes liver damage, pancreatitis with prolonged use
Interactions	*anticoagulants* – with prolonged use seems to enhance effect of warfarin *cholestyramine* – reduces the absorption of paracetamol *metaclopromide* – enhances the effect of paracetamol
Pharmacodynamic properties	antipyretic, peripherally acting analgesic

table continues

Fetal risk	epidemiological studies in human pregnancy show no ill effects
Breastfeeding	short courses only – amount secreted too small to be harmful. No controlled study data available and taken by a large number of women with no observed increase in adverse effects on breastfed infants, therefore considered safe

BP	ASPIRIN (ACETYLSALICYLIC ACID)
Proprietary	aspirin (various generic manufacturers; see BNF for advice)
Group	analgesic, non-opioid, NSAID
Uses/indications	mild to moderate pain, including headache, neuralgia, rheumatic pain, transient musculoskeletal pain, pyrexia
Type of drug	GSL (sold to the public in packs of no more than 32; pharmacists may dispense up to 100 capsules/tablets), POM
Presentation	tablets, some dispersible, suppositories
Dosage	300–900 mg 4–6-hrly to a max. 4 g daily
Route of admin	oral, p.r.
Contraindications	hypersensitivity, clotting disorders, haemophilia, asthma, angio-oedema, urticaria, rhinitis, impaired renal or hepatic function, dehydration, gastric ulceration, asthma, pregnancy, unless in very low doses on obstetrician's orders
Side effects	increased bleeding time, leading to haemorrhage, i.e. antepartum, intrapartum, postpartum, delayed onset and duration of labour (low doses are not harmful)
	mild and infrequent, gastric irritation/ulceration, hypersensitivity, bronchospasm and skin reactions in hypersensitive patients, haematuria, nervousness, dizziness, tinnitus, insomnia, rash

table continues

Interactions	*alcohol* – enhanced effect on the gut
	antacids – increased alkalinity of urine
	analgesics – concomitant admin. increases side effects
	anticoagulants – increased risk of haemorrhage (potentiates antiplatelet effect)
	antiepileptics – enhance effect of phenytoin and valproate
	corticosteroids – enhances the risk of gastrointestinal bleeding and ulceration
	metoclopramide – increases rate of absorption and therefore increased effects of aspirin
Pharmacodynamic properties	aspirin is an analgesic, antipyretic, anti-inflammatory which inhibits the synthesis of prostaglandins
Fetal risk	low-dose aspirin is not thought to have harmful effects in high doses closure of PDA in utero, persistent pulmonary hypertension, possible reduction in the amount of amniotic fluid (Little 1999, pp 629–630), not recommended after 34 weeks' gestation, kernicterus in jaundiced neonates; is also reported to be linked with fetal growth deficiency and a purpuric rash in neonates, with depression of the platelet function
Breastfeeding	potentially Reyes' syndrome, regular high doses could cause impairment of platelet function and hypoprothrombinaemia if neonatal vitamin K stores are low

BP	DICLOFENAC SODIUM
Proprietary	Voltarol® (Novartis), diclofenac sodium (non-proprietary – see BNF for manufacturers' details)
Group	analgesic, non-opioid, NSAID
Uses/indications	moderate to severe pain, musculoskeletal pain, used post LSCS, anti-inflammatory properties
Type of drug	POM
Presentation	tablets some dispersible, ampoules, suppositories
Dosage	oral: 75–150 mg daily in divided doses, preferably after food (max. 150 mg in 24 hrs)
	p.r.: 100 mg 18-hrly (max. 150 mg in 24 hrs) rarely – deep IM: 75 mg daily (max. 2 days)
Route of admin	oral, p.r., rarely deep IM
Contraindications	asthma, pregnancy, hypersensitivity to NSAIDs, cardiac, hepatic or renal impairment, clotting disorders
Side effects	uterine inertia, delayed onset and increased duration of labour, increased postpartum blood loss, coagulation disorders leading to haemorrhage, asthma, bronchospasm, gastric irritability/ulceration, rectal irritation, headache, dizziness, vertigo, abdominal pain, rash, purpura, urticaria, drowsiness, disturbances of vision, loss of sensation, malaise, fatigue and insomnia

table continues

Interactions	*analgesics* – concomitant admin. causes increased side effects
	antihypertensives – calcium channel blockers – antagonizes hypotensive effects
	β–blockers – antagonism of hypotensive effects
	methlydopa – antagonism of the hypotensive effect
	anticoagulants – *coumarins* – anticoagulant effect is increased
	heparin – increased risk of haemorrhage with IV diclofenac
	antiepileptics – phenytoin – possible enhanced effect
	zidovudine – increased risk of haematological toxicity
Pharmacodynamic properties	NSAID analgesic which inhibits prostaglandin synthesis, with antipyretic properties
Fetal risk	benefits must outweigh the risk and the lowest possible effective dose should be used; can cause closure of PDA in utero, persistent pulmonary hypertension
Breastfeeding	amount secreted too small to be harmful and evidence of risk is remote, although there are only a limited number of controlled studies in breastfeeding women

BP	CODEINE PHOSPHATE
Proprietary	codeine phosphate (non-proprietary, see BNF for details)
Group	analgesic, opioid – morphine salt
Uses/indications	mild to moderate pain, cough suppressant
Type of drug	POM, (CD – injection)
Presentation	tablets, syrup, ampoules (CD)
Dosage	oral: 30–60 mg 4-hrly (max. 240 mg daily) IM: 30–60 mg 4-hrly
Route of admin	oral, IM
Contraindications	as for morphine, raised intracranial pressure
Side effects	constipation, nausea, sedation, respiratory depression, especially cough reflex, dependence. In labour – maternal gastric stasis and increased risk of inhalation pneumonia
Interactions	as for diamorphine
Pharmacodynamic properties	codeine is a narcotic analgesic which acts via the central nervous system
Fetal risk	first trimester: inguinal hernias, cardiac, circulatory and respiratory system defects, cleft lip and palate, although not according to Little (1999, p 630)
	second trimester: alimentary tract defects
	labour: neonatal respiratory depression and withdrawal
Breastfeeding	amount secreted too small to be harmful and there are limited data available on breastfeeding women where there was no observed increase in adverse effects on breastfed infants

BP	FENTANYL
Proprietary	Sublimaze® (Janssen–Cilag Ltd), fentanyl citrate (non-proprietary, see BNF for details of manufacturers)
Group	analgesic, opioid – morphine salt
Uses/indications	enhancement of anaesthesia, i.e. epidural
Type of drug	CD, Class A, Schedule 2
Presentation	prediluted ampoules, premixed solution in polybags of 100 or 200 mL for intrathecal infusion in continuous epidurals
Dosage	50–200 µg, subsequent doses 50 µg p.r.n.
Route of admin	intrathecal (IV not used in obstetrics)
Contraindications	caution in existing respiratory depression, myasthenia gravis, known hypersensitivity to fentanyl or opioids
Side effects	respiratory depression – can be delayed, apnoea, transient hypotension, bradycardia, nausea, vomiting, itching, muscular rigidity, myoclonic movements, bradycardia, transient hypotension, urinary retention. Hypersensitivity can cause anaphylaxis
Interactions	as for morphine
Pharmacodynamic properties	a synthetic opiate with 50–100 times the clinical potency of morphine, it has a rapid onset but its duration of action is short. Its peak effect is at 30 minutes post dosage and it differs from morphine in its short duration of action and its lack of emetic effect

table continues

Fetal risk	no evidence of teratogenic or embryotoxic effects, but manufacturers advise avoidance. Crosses the placental barrier and may cause loss of fetal heart variability without fetal hypoxia, respiratory depression or withdrawal symptoms, although these may be less via intrathecal route
Breastfeeding	no controlled study data available. Although it is likely to be present in very trace amounts in breast milk there is no evidence of an increased risk of adverse effects in breastfed infants

BP	DIHYDROCODEINE TARTRATE
Proprietary	DF118 Forte® (Martindale), DHC Continus® (Napp), Dihydrocodeine (non-proprietary, see BNF for details of manufacturers)
Group	analgesic, opioid – morphine salt
Uses/indications	moderate to severe pain
Type of drug	POM, (CD – injection)
Presentation	tablets (white), elixir, ampoules (CD)
Dosage	oral: 30 mg 4–6-hrly (preferably after food), higher doses cause nausea and vomiting deep s.c. IM: 50 mg repeated 4–6-hrly
Route of admin	oral, IM, deep s.c.
Contraindications	raised intracranial pressure, respiratory difficulties
Side effects	constipation, drowsiness, respiratory depression, hypotension, dizziness, dependence; high doses cause nausea and vomiting
Interactions	as for diamorphine
Pharmacodynamic properties	dihydrocodeine is a semisynthetic narcotic analgesic with a potency between morphine and codeine which acts on the opioid receptors in the brain to reduce the patient's perception of pain and improve the psychological reaction to pain by removing associated anxiety

table continues

Fetal risk	little evidence to suggest fetal risk; however, there may be withdrawal symptoms, or respiratory depression in the neonate, and manufacturer advises use only when the benefits outweigh the risks
Breastfeeding	little evidence to suggest secretion in breast milk, but manufacturers advise avoidance

BP	PETHIDINE HYDROCHLORIDE
Proprietary	Pethidine (non-proprietary, see BNF for details of manufacturers), Pamergan P100® (Martindale)
Group	analgesic – opioid, alkaloid
Uses/indications	moderate to severe pain, obstetric analgesia
Type of drug	CD, Class A, Schedule 2, authorized by standing orders
Presentation	tablets, ampoules
Dosage	s.c./IM: 25–150 mg 4-hrly oral: 50–150 mg 4-hrly slow IV injection: 25–50 mg 4-hrly
Route of admin	IM, rarely in obstetrics – oral, s.c., slow IV injection
Contraindications	existing respiratory depression, renal impairment, pre-existing morphine addiction, compromised fetus
Side effects	nausea, vomiting, respiratory depression, convulsions after overdose, bradycardia, dependence
Interactions	as for diamorphine *antacids* – cimetidine inhibits metabolism of pethidine
Pharmacodynamic properties	as for diamorphine

table continues

Fetal risk	crosses placental barrier within 2 minutes of administration and present in amniotic fluid in 30 minutes; bradycardia, respiratory depression, withdrawal symptoms, slow excretion by neonatal liver
Breastfeeding	depresses suck reflex, as for diamorphine

BP	DIAMORPHINE HYDROCHLORIDE
Proprietary	a.k.a. heroin
Group	analgesic – morphine salt – narcotic
Uses/indications	moderate to severe pain, i.e. postoperative and labour
Type of drug	CD, Class A, Schedule 2
Presentation	tablets, powder for reconstitution
Dosage	5–10 mg 4-hrly (depending on patient size) slow IV injection 0.25–0.5 the corresponding IM dose
Route of admin	IM, oral, slow IV injection
Contraindications	existing respiratory depression, asthma, raised intracranial pressure as it affects papillary responses, phaeochromocytoma – endogenous release of histamines may stimulate catecholamine release
Side effects	gastric stasis in labour, sedation, nausea, vomiting, respiratory depression, dependence, tachycardia, hypothermia, hallucinations, mood swings, facial flushing, sweating, constipation, dizziness, miosis, confusion, urinary retention, biliary spasm, postural hypotension, vertigo, palpitations, dry mouth, urticaria, pruritus, raised intracranial pressure and rarely circulatory depression
Interactions	non-specific to diamorphine but characteristic of opioids *alcohol* – enhances the sedative effect, increases hypotension *analgesics* – enhanced effects

table continues

	antidepressants – avoid concurrent administration of MAOI or administration within 2 weeks of their discontinuation
	increases the sedative effect of tricyclics *anxiolytics and hypnotics* – enhances the sedative effect *cimetidine* – inhibits metabolism, thereby increasing the plasma concentration of the opioid *metoclopramide* – antagonism of the effect on gastrointestinal activity
Pharmacodynamic properties	narcotic analgesic acting on the central nervous system (CNS) and smooth muscle. Its predominant action is to depress the CNS, but it has stimulant actions resulting in nausea, vomiting and miosis
Fetal risk	crosses the placental barrier within 1 hr of administration, causes withdrawal symptoms, respiratory depression, meconium aspiration, intrauterine death
Breastfeeding	therapeutic doses are unlikely to affect the infant, but in dependent mothers secretion into breast milk may cause problems with withdrawal and addiction

BP	MORPHINE SULPHATE
Proprietary	Oramorph® (Boehringer Ingelheim), morphine sulphate (non-proprietary, see BNF for details of manufacturers)
Group	analgesic – narcotic
Uses/indications	postoperative pain, to potentiate epidural anaesthesia, patient-controlled analgesia systems (PCAS)
Type of drug	CD, Class A, Schedule 2 (oral – POM CD)
Presentation	oral solution, tablets, capsules, suspension, suppositories, ampoules
Dosage	IM or s.c.: 10–15 mg 4-hrly (depending on patient size, severity of pain, response and tolerance to dosage)
	slow IV injection – 0.25–0.5 of IM dose intrathecal – dosage determined by anaesthetist
	PCAS – determined by hospital protocols
	oral – rare in obstetrics: refer to BNF, but usually double IM dose, post LSCS usage is increasing, refer to BNF but typically 10–20 ml 3hrly
	p.r.: 15–30 mg 4-hrly
Route of admin	oral, IM, s.c., p.r., IV, intrathecal
Contraindications	renal or hepatic impairment, respiratory depression, asthma, raised intracranial pressure (affects papillary responses), phaeochromocytoma

table continues

Side effects	as for diamorphine NB: postoperative patients should be observed closely for delayed or rebound respiratory depression as well as other side effects
Interactions	as for diamorphine
Pharmacodynamic properties	morphine is a narcotic analgesic obtained from opium and which acts on the central nervous system and smooth muscle
Fetal risk	as for diamorphine
Breastfeeding	therapeutic doses unlikely to affect the infant and so it is considered moderately safe

BP	HYOSCINE BUTYLBROMIDE
Proprietary	Buscopan® (Boehringer Ingelheim)
Group	antimuscarinics
Uses/indications	gastrointestinal smooth muscle spasm, irritable bowel, diverticular disease, dysmenorrhoea
Type of drug	POM, (GSL – sold to the public provided a single dose does not exceed 20 mg and the daily dose of 80 mg; packs are restricted to 240 mg max.)
Presentation	tablets, ampoules
Dosage	oral: 20 mg q.d.s. IM, IV injection: 20 mg repeated after 30 minutes if required
Route of admin	oral, IM, IV injection
Contraindications	myasthenia gravis, paralytic ileus
Side effects	constipation, transient bradycardia followed by tachycardia, palpitations, arrhythmias, urinary urgency and retention, photophobia, dry mouth, flushing and skin dryness; rarely–nausea, vomiting, giddiness, confusion
Interactions	*alcohol* – enhances sedative effect of hyoscine *antidepressants* – tricyclics have increased side effects *antihistamines* – increase the antimuscarinic side effects *MAOIs* – increased antimuscarinic effects *phenothiazines* – chlorpromazine increases the antimuscarinic side effects

table continues

Pharmacodynamic properties	antispasmodic agent that relaxes the smooth muscle of the organs of the abdominal and pelvic cavities and acts on the intramural parasympathetic ganglia of these organs
Fetal risk	animal studies show teratogenicity, but there are no controlled studies in pregnant women. Not recommended by manufacturer unless benefits outweigh the risks
Breastfeeding	not recommended by manufacturer, but considered moderately safe as there are no observed increases in adverse effects in breastfed infants

Chapter **4**

Antibiotics

These are produced by certain bacteria or fungi that interfere with or prevent the growth of other bacteria/fungi. They are used in infection or as prophylaxis, e.g. in cases of spontaneous rupture of membranes longer than 24 hours, or in lower-segment caesarean section.

The student should be aware of:

- Causes and transmission of infection
- Causal organisms of infection and their laboratory identification
- The symptoms and progression of infection
- The importance of bacterial culture and sensitivity
- The ingestion, uptake, action and excretion of the prescribed drug
- The Royal College of Obstetricians and Gynaecologists' (2000) protocol for antibiotic prophylaxis in patients with diagnosed heart disease, heart murmurs or prosthetic heart valves: at the commencement of labour – IV ampicillin 1 g plus gentamicin 120 mg, then 500 mg oral ampicillin 6-hourly. In penicillin-sensitive patients vancomycin 1 g replaces ampicillin.

References

Briggs GG, Freeman RK, Yaffe SJ. Drugs in pregnancy and lactation: a reference guide to fetal and neonatal risk, 3rd edn. Baltimore: Williams & Wilkins, 1990

British Medical Association and the Royal Pharmaceutical Society of Great Britain. British national formulary. No 43 March 2002. Bath: Bath Press, 2002

Hale T. Medications and mothers' milk, 9th edn. USA: Pharmasoft Publications, 2000

Hopkins SJ. Drugs and pharmacology for nurses, 13th edn. Edinburgh: Churchill Livingstone, 1999

Little BB. Medication during pregnancy. In: James DK, Steer PJ, Weiner CP, Gonik B, eds. High risk pregnancy: management options, 2nd edn. London: WB Saunders, 1999; 620–621

Roth C. Sexually transmissible and reproductive tract infection in pregnancy. In: Bennett VR, Brown LK, eds. Myles textbook for midwives, 13th edn. Edinburgh: Churchill Livingstone, 1999; 329–350

Sampson JE, Gravett MG. Other infectious conditions in pregnancy. In: James DK, Steer PJ, Weiner CP, Gonik B, eds. High risk pregnancy: management options, 2nd edn. London: WB Saunders, 1999; 559–598

Stockley IH (ed) Drug interactions, 5th edn. London: Pharmaceutical Press, 1999

SPC from the eMC, Monotrim Tablets®, Solvay Healthcare Ltd, updated on the eMC 14/09/01

SPC from the eMC, Genticin® injectable Roche Products Ltd, updated on the eMC 26/11/01

SPC from the eMC, Cidomycin®, adult injectable 80 mg/2 ml, Hoechst Marion Roussel Ltd, updated on the eMC 23/08/01

SPC from the eMC, Erythrocin®, Abbot Laboratories Ltd, updated on the eMC 23/08/01

SPC from the eMC, Floxapen® capsules, syrup, vials for injection, SmithKline Beecham Pharmaceuticals, updated on the eMC 25/03/02

SPC from the eMC, Velosef® capsules 250 mg, syrup 250 mg/5 mL, Velosef for injections, ER Squibb and Sons Ltd, updated on the eMC 14/08/01

SPC from the eMC, Amoxil®, SmithKline Beecham Pharmaceuticals, updated on the eMC 16/08/01

SPC from the eMC, Crystapen®, Britannia Pharmaceuticals Ltd, updated on the eMC 30/08/01

SPC from the eMC, Penbritin® vials 500 mg, capsules 250 mg, SmithKline Beecham Pharmaceuticals, updated on the eMC 05/08/01, and 10/08/01

SPC from the eMC, Augmentin® IV, tablets and powder, SmithKline Beecham Pharmaceuticals, updated on the eMC 09/07/02

SPC from the eMC, Flagyll®, tablets and suspension, Hawgreen Ltd, updated on the eMC 30/08/01

SPC from the eMC, Flagyll® suppositories, Hawgreen Ltd, updated on the eMC 29/08/01

SPC from the eMC, Flagyll® injection 100 mL, Hawgreen Ltd, updated on the eMC 14/01/02

Tomlinson MW, Colton DB. Cardiac disease. In: James DK, Steer PJ, Weiner CP, Gonik B, eds. High risk pregnancy: management options, 2nd edn. London: WB Saunders, 1999; 685–707

BP	METRONIDAZOLE
Proprietary	Flagyl® (Hawgreen Ltd) (Aventis Pharma), Metrolyl® (Lagap), Flagyl® injection (Rhone-Poulenc Rorer), metronidazole (non-proprietary, see BNF for details)
Group	antimicrobial
Uses/indications	treatment of anaerobic infection with a wide range of activity, prophylaxis in surgery, clostridium, *Trichomonas vaginalis*, puerperal sepsis, bacterial vaginosis, gingivitis
Type of drug	POM
Presentation	tablets, suspension, suppositories, pre-prepared IV injections and infusions
Dosage	oral: stat 800 mg then 400–500 mg t.d.s. IV: 500 mg t.d.s. LSCS 400 mg t.d.s. (500 mg at intubation) p.r.: 1 g t.d.s. for 3 days max. then 1 g b.d. treatment of bacterial vaginosis as for oral or 2 g single dose
Route of admin	oral, p.r., IV, IM
Contraindications	in pregnancy and breastfeeding avoid high dosage, avoid alcohol, known hypersensitivity to metronidazole
Side effects	unpleasant taste in mouth, furry tongue, nausea, vomiting, rashes, headache, drowsiness, dizziness, dark urine and very rarely angio-oedema

table continues

Interactions	*alcohol* – disulfiram-like reaction – avoid during treatment and for 48 hours post course *antacids* – cimetidine inhibits the metabolism of metronidazole *anticoagulants* – enhances the effect of warfarin but no interaction with heparin *antiepileptics* – inhibits the metabolism of phenytoin phenobarbitone accelerates metabolism of metronidazole *oestrogens* – reduces the effect of the combined oral contraceptive pill
Pharmacodynamic properties	antimicrobial effective against a wide range of infections with antiprotozoal and antibacterial actions
Fetal risk	avoid high-dose regimens; use in first trimester can cause midline facial defects, cardiac defects, genital defects and limb defects, but has been used with little effect in last two trimesters
Breastfeeding	significant amounts secreted, avoid large single doses

BP	ERYTHROMYCIN
Proprietary	Erythrocin® (Abbot Laboratories Ltd), Erymax® (Elan), erythromycin (non-proprietary, see BNF for details)
Group	antibiotic, macrolide
Uses/indications	used in penicillin-sensitive clients, penicillin-resistant organisms, syphilis, chlamydia, gonorrhoea, respiratory infection, treatment of infection sensitive to erythromycin, prophylaxis in management of pre-term rupture of membranes. Also in patients requiring antibiotic cover for heart disease and heart valves who are sensitive to penicillin
Type of drug	POM
Presentation	tablets, capsules, powder for reconstitution, granules, suspension
Dosage	1–2 g/day in even doses, depending on the severity of infection oral: 250–500 mg q.d.s.or 0.5–1 g b.d. syphilis/chlamydia: 500 mg q.d.s. for 14 days IV: 25–50 mg/kg daily or 1–2 g in 6 even doses
Route of admin	oral, IV
Contraindications	hypersensitivity, hepatic dysfunction
Side effects	nausea, vomiting, diarrhoea, fever skin eruptions, urticaria, rashes, cardiac arrhythmias; in large doses: reversible hearing loss, hepatic dysfunction, thrombophlebitis following IV, allergic response rare with mild anaphylaxis

table continues

Interactions	*anticoagulants* – effect of warfarin enhanced *antihistamines* – inhibits the metabolism of terfenadine, causing dangerous cardiac arrhythmias *cisapride* – can cause cardiotoxicity and arrhythmias *ergotamines* – acute ergot toxicity, rapid peripheral vasospasm and dysaesthesia *theophylline* – inhibition of metabolism of theophylline
Pharmacodynamic properties	antimicrobial which attaches to a subunit of susceptible organisms and suppresses protein synthesis, destroying cell wall stability and making them vulnerable to attack. Active against both Gram-positive and Gram-negative bacteria, mycoplasms, treponema, chlamydia and gonorrhoea
Fetal risk	crosses the placental barrier but not in appreciable quantities; fetal concentrations have found to be low, with no reports of congenital defects located; however, Little (1999) advises that if used to treat maternal syphilitic infection the infant will be born with congenital syphilis, therefore consider alternative treatment for maternal disease
Breastfeeding	only secreted in small amounts in breast milk – considered safe with no ill effects reported, although manufacturers advise avoidance

BP	CEPHRADINE (CEFRADINE)
Proprietary	Velosef® (Squibb), cephradine (non-proprietary, see BNF for details)
Group	antibiotic – cephalosporin
Uses/indications	against both Gram-positive and -negative bacteria, prophylaxis with LSCS, UTI, respiratory infections
Type of drug	POM
Presentation	capsules, syrup, powder for reconstitution
Dosage	oral: 250–500 mg 6–8-hrly or 0.5–1 g b.d. IM, IV: 500 mg–1 g q.d.s. given over 3–5 minutes
Route of admin	oral, IM, IV
Contraindications	renal dysfunction, known hypersensitivity to cephalosporins, caution in penicillin hypersensitivity
Side effects	nausea, diarrhoea and hypersensitivity – usually mild, headache, dizziness, dyspnoea
Interactions	nil specific to cephradine: *anticoagulants* – effect of warfarin enhanced *uricosurics* – excretion is reduced by probenecid *oestrogens* – reduces the effect of the combined oral contraceptive pill

table continues

Pharmacodynamic properties	broad-spectrum bactericidal drug active against Gram-positive organisms, e.g. staphylococci, streptococci, *Streptococcus pyogenes, Streptococcus pneumoniae*, and Gram-negative organisms such as *E. coli, Haemophilus influenzae*, salmonella. Highly active against penicillinase-producing staphylococci. e.g. *S. aureus*
Fetal risk	no reports of congenital defects located, although manufacturers advise safety not established
Breastfeeding	considered safe, although manufacturers advise caution – as for amoxycillin

BP	FLUCLOXACILLIN SODIUM
Proprietary	Floxapen® (SmithKline Beecham), flucloxacillin (non-proprietary, see BNF for details)
Group	antibiotic, penicillinase-resistant penicillin
Uses/indications	against β-lactamase resistant microbes, including *S. aureus* and streptococci, prophylaxis in surgery
Type of drug	POM
Presentation	capsules, syrup, powder for reconstitution
Dosage	oral: 250–500 mg t.d.s. (30–60 min before food) IV/infusion: 250 mg–2 g q.d.s. IM: 250–500 mg q.d.s. (according to severity of infection) prophylaxis: 1–2 g IV at induction of anaesthesia, then 500 mg q.d.s. IM or IV for up to 72 hrs
Route of admin	oral, IM, IV/infusion
Contraindications	penicillin and/or cephalosporin hypersensitivity, sodium-restricted diet, renal or hepatic impairment
Side effects	anaphylaxis – uncommon and usually mild and transitory, diarrhoea, rash, indigestion, rarely hepatic impairment, reversible neutropenia, thrombocytopenia
Interactions	*contraceptives* – reduces contraceptive effect

table continues

Pharmacodynamic properties	narrow-spectrum penicillin which is not inactivated by staphylococcal lactamases. It acts on the synthesis of the bacterial wall and exerts a bactericidal effect on streptococci, including *Neisseria* and *Clostridia*, but not MRSA
Fetal risk	animal studies show no teratogenicity but manufacturer advises that it should be withheld unless considered essential
Breastfeeding	considered safe, but as for amoxycillin

BP	CO-AMOXICLAV (COMPOUND OF AMOXYCILLIN AS A SODIUM SALT AND CLAVULANIC ACID)
Proprietary	Augmentin® (SmithKline Beecham)
Group	antibiotic, broad-spectrum penicillinase
Uses/indications	against bacteria resistant to amoxycillin, i.e. *S. aureus*, *E. coli*, gonorrhoea, β-lactamase infection, UTI, abdominal infection, cellulitis, prophylaxis at LSCS or MRP
Type of drug	POM
Presentation	tablets, dispersible tablets, suspension, powder for reconstitution
Dosage	oral: 375 mg (250 mg expressed as amoxycillin) t.d.s.; 625 mg (500 mg) t.d.s in severe infection IV: 600 mg–1.2 g t.d.s.
Route of admin	oral, IV, IV infusion
Contraindications	penicillin and/or cephalosporin hypersensitivity, jaundice/hepatic dysfunction
Side effects	nausea, diarrhoea, rashes, rarely hepatic impairment, hypersensitivity, CNS effects – rare, vaginal itching, soreness and discharge
Interactions	nil specific *anticoagulants* – may prolong bleeding time and prothrombin time *contraceptives* – reduces contraceptive effect

table continues

Pharmacodynamic properties	resistance to antibiotics is caused by bacterial enzymes destroying it before it is able to act on the pathogen. The clavulanate anticipates this and blocks β-lactamase enzymes in organisms sensitive to amoxycillin. Co-amoxiclav has a rapid bactericidal effect
Fetal risk	animal studies with oral and parenteral administration show no teratogenicity, but manufacturers advise avoidance in the first trimester and use thereafter only when considered essential
	second/third trimesters – in a single study women with preterm premature rupture of membranes given Augmentin for prophylaxis against infection found an association with necrotizing enterocolitis in the neonate (SPC – Augmentin 9/07/02)
Breastfeeding	trace quantities excreted but considered safe – as for amoxycillin

BP	AMOXYCILLIN
Proprietary	Amoxil® (SmithKline Beecham)
Group	antibiotic, broad-spectrum penicillinase
Uses/indications	broad spectrum, used against Gram-positive and Gram-negative bacteria, except pseudomonas, respiratory infections, UTI, gonorrhoea, puerperal sepsis, routine prophylaxis in clients with heart valves or heart disease concomitant with gentamicin, bacterial endocarditis
Type of drug	POM
Presentation	capsules, dispersible tablets, sachets, powder for reconstitution
Dosage	oral: 250–500 mg t.d.s. IM: 500 mg t.d.s. IV: 500 mg t.d.s. to 1 g q.d.s. in severe infection prophylaxis with heart valves etc.: 1 g IV then 500 mg 6 hrs later
Route of admin	oral, IM, IV/infusion
Contraindications	penicillin hypersensitivity
Side effects	mild diarrhoea, indigestion, rash, rarely anaphylaxis – usually mild
Interactions	*anticoagulants* – causes prolonged prothrombin time *contraceptives* – reduces contraceptive effect *uricosurics* – excretion reduced with concomitant admin. of probenecid – used in treatment of gonorrhoea

table continues

Pharmacodynamic properties	broad-spectrum antibiotic with rapid bactericidal effects, which has the safety profile of penicillin
Fetal risk	nil known, no reports of toxicity in animal or human studies, but manufacturers advise benefits should outweigh the risks
Breastfeeding	considered safe but modifies the bowel flora and can cause sensitization; interferes with culture results if an infection screen is required

BP	TRIMETHOPRIM
Proprietary	Monotrim® (Solvay Healthcare Ltd)
Group	antimicrobial – sulphonamide
Uses/indications	treatment of sensitive organisims, UTI, URTI, prophylaxis against UTI
Type of drug	POM
Presentation	tablets, suspension, injection
Dosage	oral: 200 mg b.d.
	IV injection/infusion: 200 mg b.d.
	prophylaxis: 200 mg
Route of admin	oral, IV
Contraindications	pregnancy, hypersensitivity to trimethoprim, blood dyscrasias, renal insufficiency or impairment
Side effects	nausea, vomiting, rash – mild and reversible, allergic reactions, including anaphylaxis
Interactions	*anticonvulsants* – half-life of phenytoin is increased, antifolate effect enhanced *anticoagulants* – enhanced anticoagulant effect *oestrogens* – reduces the effect of the combined oral contraceptive pill
Pharmacodynamic properties	antimicrobial which works by selective inhibition of bacterial dihydrofolate reductase. It is effective against both Gram-positive and -negative aerobic organisms, including *E. coli, Proteus, Klebsiella, S. aureus, Strep. faecalis* and

table continues

	pneumoniae, Haemophilus influenzae, but NOT *Neisseria, Pseudomonas aeruginosa, Treponema pallidum* or anaerobes
Fetal risk	first trimester: teratogen – as a folate antagonist manufacturers advise avoidance as can cause transient hyperbilirubinaemia in the neonate (Little 1999)
Breastfeeding	excreted in small amounts but considered moderately safe in the short term

BP	GENTAMICIN
Proprietary	Gentacin® (Roche), Cidomycin® (Hoechst Marion Roussel)
Group	broad-spectrum aminoglycoside antibiotic
Uses/indications	systemic infection, prophylaxis during labour for patients with heart valves/heart disease, UTI, chest infection
Type of drug	POM
Presentation	ampoules
Dosage	3–4 mg/kg body weight daily in divided doses (e.g. 80 mg 8-hrly in patients over 60 kg, or 60 mg 8-hrly in those under 60 kg)
Route of admin	IM, IV slow injection, IV infusion
Contraindications	hypersensitivity, myasthenia gravis, renal impairment
Side effects	toxicity – renal toxicity reversible after withdrawal. Vestibular hearing loss/damage, hypersensitivity
Interactions	avoid concomitant use with ototoxic and nephrotoxic drugs *muscle relaxants* – enhances the muscle relaxant effect *oestrogens* – may reduce the effect of the combined oral contraceptive pill
Pharmacodynamic properties	bactericidal aminoglycoside that acts by inhibiting protein synthesis, acting on the integrity of the plasma membrane and metabolism of ribonucleic acid

table continues

Fetal risk	safety is not established and it crosses the placental barrier second/third trimester – probably low risk but potentially may cause deafness
Breastfeeding	present in breast milk, and although unlikely to cause problems the manufacturers advise avoidance

BP	BENZYLPENICILLIN
Proprietary	(Penicillin G) Crystapen® (Britannia)
Group	antibiotic – penicillinase
Uses/indications	streptococcal infection, i.e. throat infection, ear infection, pneumonia, treatment of gonorrhoea
Type of drug	POM
Presentation	vials of powder for reconstitution
Dosage	IM, IV injection or IV infusion: 2.4–4.8 g in four divided doses (available in 600 mg and 1200 mg doses equivalent to 1 and 2 megaunits)
Route of admin	IM, IV injection/infusion
Contraindications	hypersensitivity to penicillin
Side effects	hypersensitivity – urticaria, fever, joint pain, rashes, anaphylaxis, diarrhoea, thrombocytopenia, neutropenia, haemolytic anaemia – in high doses
Interactions	nil specific
oestrogens – reduces the effect of combined oral contraceptive pill
Pharmacodynamic properties	bacteriostatic with bactericidal activities against Gram-negative coli. It is inactivated by gastric acid and is therefore best given IV or by injection
Fetal risk	nil reported
Breastfeeding	no data available from controlled studies in breastfeeding women, although it is considered safe

BP	AMPICILLIN
Proprietary	Ampicillin (non-proprietary, see BNF for details), Penbritin® (SmithKline Beecham)
Group	broad-spectrum antibiotic, penicillin
Uses/indications	UTI, ear infection, sinusitis, bronchitis, *Haemophilus influenzae*, salmonella, meningococcal disease, listerial meningitis
Type of drug	POM
Presentation	capsules, suspension, vials for injection
Dosage	oral: 0.25–1 g q.d.s. (taken 30 minutes before food) IM, IV/IVI: 500 mg 4–6-hrly
Route of admin	oral, IM, IV
Contraindications	hypersensitivity to penicillin, history of renal impairment, caution with erythematous rash
Side effects	GI disturbances, rashes, hypersensitivity – anaphylaxis
Interactions	*antibiotics* – concurrent use of bacteriostatic drugs can interfere with the bactericidal action of ampicillin *anticoagulants* – INR may be altered by course of broad-spectrum antibiotics *oestrogens* – reduces the effectiveness of combined oral contraceptive pill
Pharmacodynamic properties	broad-spectrum antibiotic indicated in the treatment of a wide range of bacterial infections caused by ampicillin-sensitive organisms

table continues

Fetal risk	manufacturer advises no risk
Breastfeeding	trace amounts excreted into breast milk, but there are no adequate data about use during lactation, no advice re avoidance

Chapter 5

Anticoagulants

These are substances used to prevent blood clotting.
The student should be aware of:

- Factors predisposing to thromboembolism
- Local protocols for management of thromboembolism
- The antagonist for such treatment and its availability
- Factors involved in the mechanism of blood clotting, and the criteria used to determine which is the most appropriate anticoagulant
- Conditions requiring treatment with anticoagulants
- Maternal and fetal sequelae of such treatment
- The effects of progesterone on the circulatory system.
  Heparin antagonist: protamine sulphate
  Warfarin antagonist: vitamin K and plasma

References

Briggs GG, Freeman RK, Yaffe SJ. Drugs in pregnancy and lactation: a reference guide to fetal and neonatal risk, 3rd edn. Baltimore: Williams & Wilkins, 1990

British Medical Association and the Royal Pharmaceutical Society of Great Britain. British national formulary. No 43 March 2002. Bath: Bath Press, 2002

de Sweit M. Thromboembolic disease. In: James DK, Steer PJ, Wiener CP, Gonik B, eds. High risk pregnancy: management options, 2nd edn. London: WB Saunders, 1999; 901–909

Hale T. Medications and mothers' milk, 9th edn. USA: Pharmasoft Publications, 2000

Hopkins SJ. Drugs and pharmacology for nurses, 13th edn. Edinburgh: Churchill Livingstone, 1999

Little BB. Medication during pregnancy. In: James DK, Steer PJ, Wiener CP, Gonik B, eds. High risk pregnancy: management options, 2nd edn. London: WB Saunders, 1999; 617–638

Royal College of Obstetricians and Gynaecologists. Thromboembolic disease in pregnancy and the puerperium: acute management. Clinical Greentop Guidelines No.28, April 2001

SPC from the eMC, Marevan®, Goldshield Pharmaceuticals Ltd, updated on the eMC 14/05/02

SPC from the eMC, Innohep® 20 000 IU/mL and Innohep syringe 20 000 IU/mL, Leo Laboratories Ltd, updated on the eMC 15/03/02

SPC from the eMC, Fragmin® 10 000 IU, 12 500 IU, 15 000 IU, 18 000 IU syringes, Pharmacia, updated on the eMC 12/07/01

SPC from the eMC, Clexane® injection, Rhone-Poulenc Rorer Ltd, update on the eMC 10/07/02

SPC from the eMC, Calciparine®, Sanofi Synthelabo, updated on the eMC 21/08/01

SPC from the eMC, Prosulf® protamine sulphate injection BP, C.P. Pharmaceuticals Ltd, updated on the eMC 28/08/01

SPC from the eMC, Konakion MM®, Roche Products Ltd, updated on the eMC 06/08/01

Stockley IH (ed) Drug interactions. London: Pharmaceutical Press, 1999

www.facs.org/dept/jacs/articles/sumpio/html – the pharmacodynamic properties of heparin

www.people.vcu.edu/~urdesai/hep.htm – the pharmacodynamic properties of heparin

www.tigc.org/eguidelines/heparin/htm – the pharmacodynamic properties of heparin

BP	HEPARIN (AS SODIUM OR CALCIUM SALT)
Proprietary	Calciprine® (Sanofi Synthelabo), Monoparin® (CP), Minihep® (Leo)
Group	anticoagulant, parenteral
Uses/indications	treatment of DVT, pulmonary embolism, thromboembolism-susceptible clients, prophylaxis in emergency LSCS
Type of drug	POM
Presentation	preloaded syringes, ampoules
Dosage	IV: 5000 units loading dose and then continuous infusion of 15–25 units/kg/hr adjusted by laboratory monitoring (severe PE: loading dose 10 000 units)
	s.c.: after LSCS 5000 b.d. until ambulant
	during pregnancy: 5–10 000 units b.d. –monitoring required
	DVT: 15 000 units b.d.
Route of admin	s.c., IV
Contraindications	Haemorrhagic disorders, including heparin-induced thrombocytopenia, cerebral aneurysm, cerebral vascular accident/cerebral haemorrhage, severe hypertension, peptic ulcer, haemophilia, liver disease, major trauma, hypersensitivity, threatened abortion
Side effects	haemorrhage, including placental sites, thrombocytopenia hypersensitivity, bruising and haematoma formation. Prolonged use is associated with osteoporosis

table continues

Interactions	nil specific *anticoagulants* – concomitant use enhances effects: use caution when transferring to oral anticoagulants *antihistamines* – decreases the anticoagulant effect *aspirin* – antiplatelet effect enhanced by heparin *diclofenac* – increased risk of haemorrhage (with IV diclofenac) *GTN* – the excretion of heparin is increased by the GTN decreasing the anticoagulant effect *NSAIDs I.V.* – possible increased risk of bleeding
Pharmacodynamic properties	a naturally occurring anticoagulant that is synthesized and excreted by mast cells in the body. It acts by forming a complex with antithrombin, catalysing the inhibition of several activated blood coagulation factors and thrombin. This prevents the conversion of fibrinogen to fibrin, which is crucial for clot formation. The onset of action is immediate and it is most commonly used for the prevention and treatment of venous and arterial thromboembolism
Fetal risk	available data suggest there is no risk to fetus or neonate
Breastfeeding	not excreted in breast milk
NB:	Discontinue use prior to peridural anaesthesia, i.e. 8–12 hrs; can cause spinal haematoma or permanent paralysis

table continues

OVERDOSE	indicated by haemorrhage

APTT and platelet count should be determined. Minor haemorrhage rarely requires specific treatment and decreasing or delaying subsequent doses of heparin should be sufficient. Major haemorrhage: the anticoagulant effect is reduced immediately by 1% protamine sulphate, but caution is required as protamine also has an anticoagulant effect. A single dose should never exceed 50 mg

IV injection of protamine can cause a sudden fall in blood pressure, bradycardia, dyspnoea and transitory flushing, but this can be avoided or decreased by slow and careful administration

BP	WARFARIN SODIUM
Proprietary	Marevan® (Goldshield Pharm. Ltd), warfarin (non-proprietary, see BNF for details)
Group	anticoagulant – oral
Uses/indications	prophylaxis after prosthetic heart valve surgery, DVT, pulmonary embolism, and transient ischaemic accidents
Type of drug	POM
Presentation	tablets, white 0.5 mg, brown 1 mg, blue 3 mg, pink 5 mg
Dosage	refer to pharmacist or BNF; usually 3–10 mg daily
Route of admin	Oral
Contraindications	**pregnancy,** but may be used between 16 and 36 weeks' gestation if heparin not available and risks of thrombosis outweigh the risk to the fetus; peptic ulcer, severe hypertension, bacterial endocarditis, haemorrhage, use within 24 hrs of surgery or labour – caution if at all
Side effects	haemorrhage, nausea, transient alopecia, hypersensitivity, fall in haematocrit, purple toes, liver dysfunction, pancreatitis
Interactions	*alcohol* – enhanced effects with large alcohol doses *antacids* – cimetidine inhibits the metabolism and enhances the effect of warfarin

table continues

aspirin – increased risk of haemorrhage
– antiplatelet effect
antibiotics – cefalosporins, macrolides,
erythromycin and metronidazole,
sulphonamides, trimethoprim – possible
enhanced coagulant effect
penicillins – possible alteration of INR
antidepressants – SSRIs – anticoagulant
effect increased
dextropropoxyphene – anticoagulant
effect enhanced
paracetamol – theoretical increased risk
of bleeds with prolonged use
cholestyramine – enhanced anticoagulant
effect
barbiturates – metabolism of warfarin
increased, therefore diminishes the
anticoagulant effect
antiepileptics – carbamazepine and
phenobarbitone – diminishes the
anticoagulant effect
phenytoin – both enhances and
diminishes warfarin's effect
sodium valproate – enhanced
anticoagulant effect
oral contraceptive – diminished
contraceptive effect
NSAIDs – enhanced anticoagulant effect
mefenamic acid – enhances
anticoagulant effect
progestogen – antagonism of
anticoagulant effect

table continues

Pharmacodynamic properties	synthetic anticoagulant of the coumarin series. It acts by inhibiting the formation of active clotting factors II, VII, IX and X. An effective PT time can be achieved in 24–36 hrs post initial dose, max. 36–48 hrs, and this therapeutic PT is maintained for 48 hrs after stopping drug
Fetal risk	fetal teratogen, causes multiple disorders and malformations; should be stopped pre conception or within 6 weeks' gestation (see above). Haemorrhage in fetus and placenta in all trimesters, postnatal developmental delay
Breastfeeding	not excreted in breast milk; theoretical risk of haemorrhage, especially with vitamin K deficiency, but considered safe

BP	PROTAMINE SULPHATE
Proprietary	Prosulf® (CP) protamine sulphate (non-proprietary, see BNF)
Group	heparin antagonist
Uses/indications	reversal of the actions of heparin
Type of drug	POM
Presentation	ampoules
Dosage	see BNF and manufacturers' guidelines. *In brief:* 1 mg neutralizes 100 units heparin (mucus) or 80 units (lung) within 15 minutes of administration; if longer less is required as heparin is rapidly excreted. Max. dose 50 mg in 10 minutes. Should be monitored by activated partial prothrombin time (APPT) or other clotting test 5–10 minutes after administration; further doses may be required as protamine is cleared more rapidly than heparin, especially LMWH
Route of admin	Slow IV injection
Contraindications	hypersensitivity to protamine, caution in those receiving protamine insulin preparation, i.e. isophane insulin, fish allergy
Side effects	flushing, nausea, vomiting, hypotension, bradycardia; if overdosed then acts as an anticoagulant
Interactions	caution in those receiving isophane insulins – hypersensitivity

table continues

Pharmacodynamic properties	a potent antidote to heparin but the precise mechanism is unknown. It is assumed that the strongly basic protamine combines with the strongly acid heparin to produce a stable salt that has no anticoagulant activity
Fetal risk	insufficient information available – no animal or human studies have been carried out
Breastfeeding	no data available – as for fetal risk

BP	PHYTOMENADIONE (VITAMIN K)
Proprietary	Konakion® MM (Roche Products Ltd)
Group	warfarin antagonist
Uses/indications	prevention and treatment of haemorrhage
Type of Drug.	POM
Presentation	tablets, ampoules
Dosage	refer to manufacturers' guidelines: life-threatening haemorrhage: 5 mg slow IV injection plus plasma (factors II, IX, VII if available)
	less severe haemorrhage: withhold warfarin and consider 0.5–2 mg slow IV injection
	repeat PT levels 3 hrs post dose and if not responsive then repeat dose – not more than 40 mg in 24 hrs
Route of admin	very slow IV injection, oral, IM
Contraindications	no data available
Side effects	no data available
Interactions	*anticoagulants* – antagonism of the anticoagulant effect
Pharmacodynamic properties	synthetic vitamin K. Vitamin K is essential for the formation of prothrombin, factor VII, factor IX, and factor X. Without vitamin K there is a tendency to haemorrhage
Fetal risk	poor placental transfer, no risk data available
Breastfeeding	maternal doses – not enough information available to allow classification as safe drug. Large maternal doses of anticoagulants may require neonatal vitamin K prophylaxis

Low molecular weight heparin (LMWH) acts slightly differently to unfractionated heparin (UFH). It is essential to have an understanding of the coagulation cascade in order to understand how and why heparin is an anticoagulant. The advantage of LMWH over UFH is in its action: the actions of UFH are influenced by its binding to plasma protein, endothelial cell surfaces, macrophages and other acute-phase reactants in the anticoagulant cascade. The LMWH has decreased binding to non-anticoagulant-related plasma proteins. The anticoagulant response is predictable and reproducible, with no need for laboratory monitoring, and it is given on a weight-adjusted basis. It has a high bioavailability of 90% versus the 30% of UFH, and has a longer plasma half-life of 4–6 hours versus the 0.5–1 hour of UFH. There is less inhibition of platelet function and potentially less bleeding risk, although this is unproven. There is a lower incidence of thrombocytopenia and thrombosis as there is less interaction with platelet factor 4 (*www.cardiology.utmb.edu*).

Below are some of the LMWH and their dosages, properties, pregnancy and breastfeeding risks:

OVERDOSE: protamine sulphate only partially neutralizes these drugs, so use with caution and consider the side effects of protamine carefully.

BP	DALTEPARIN SODIUM
Proprietary	Fragmin® (Pharmacia)
Group	LMWH
Presentation	single-dose syringe, ampoules,
Dosage	PE/DVT: s.c., depending on body weight: 69–82 kg 15 000 units daily, 83 kg and over 18 000 units daily oral anticoagulants can be used concomitantly until therapeutic range is achieved (usually 5 days)
Route of admin	s.c.
Pharmacodynamic properties	porcine-derived sodium heparin and antithrombotic agent with the ability to potentiate the inhibition of Factor Xa and thrombin by antithrombin. This ability is relatively higher than disruption of the plasma clotting line (expressed as APTT), therefore compared to UFH dalteparin has fewer adverse effects on platelet function and adhesion, thus giving only minimal effects on primary haemostasis
Fetal risk	as for heparin
Breastfeeding	as for heparin

BP	ENOXOPARIN
Proprietary	Clexane® (Rhone-Poulenc Rorer)
Group	LMWH
Presentation	single-dose syringe
Dosage	PE/DVT: s.c. 1.5 mg/kg every 24 hrs for at least 5 days or until oral anticoagulation is established (150 units/kg/day)
	prophylaxis: moderate risk 20 mg (2000 units) daily for 7–10 days
	high risk: 40 mg (4000 units) daily
	medical clients: 40 mg (4000 units) daily for 6 days or until ambulant
Route of admin	s.c.
Pharmacodynamic properties	LMWH with antithrombotic activity. There is a greater rate of this than with UFH, and at the recommended dose it does not significantly alter platelet aggregation, the binding of fibrinogen to platelets, or global clotting tests such as APTT and PT time
Fetal risk	no evidence of risk in the second trimester but no information on the first and third trimesters. As there are no adequate controlled studies it is not advised for use unless there is no safe alternative
Breastfeeding	excretion into breast milk is unlikely but manufacturer advises avoidance

BP	TINZEPARIN SODIUM
Proprietary	Innohep® (Leo)
Group	LMWH
Presentation	single-dose syringe, ampoules
Dosage	caution: can cause bronchospasm and shock in asthmatics
	PE/DVT: s.c. 175 units/kg daily for 6 days or until oral anticoagulation is established after epidural/spinal anaesthesia: delay subsequent dose by at least 4 hrs
Route of admin	s.c.
Pharmacodynamic properties	antithrombotic agent which acts by inhibiting the action of several activated coagulation factors, especially Factor Xa
Fetal risk	no transplacental transmission has been found in the second trimester, but studies in rats show low birthweight, therefore the manufacturer advises avoidance
Breastfeeding	no evidence of excretion found, but manufacturer advises avoidance

Chapter 6

Anticonvulsants

These are drugs used to arrest or prevent fits or seizures. The benefits of treatment should outweigh the risk to the fetus and efforts should be made to use the single most effective drug, as teratogenicity increases with the number of drugs used.

This drug group inhibits the uptake of folic acid, and therefore any supplements given may need to be continued throughout pregnancy.

Magnesium sulphate is also an anticonvulsant used in the emergency treatment of eclampsia – see chapter on emergency drugs.

The student should be aware of:

- Conditions which require anticonvulsant therapy
- Local protocols for anticonvulsant therapy
- Recognition of fits, seizures and convulsions
- Resuscitative techniques and care of affected clients
- Maternal and fetal sequelae of absorption of these preparations.

INTERACTIONS

Phenytoin

Alcohol – high intake increases plasma phenytoin levels; chronic abuse decreases serum levels

Analgesics – NSAIDs increase the plasma phenytoin concentration

Antacids – reduce the absorption of phenytoin; cimetidine decreases the metabolism of phenytoin and therefore increases its plasma concentration

Antibiotics – metronidazole increases the plasma phenytoin concentration; plasma concentration and antifolate effect increased by trimoxazole and trimethoprim

Anticoagulants – probably reduce the effect of warfarin

Antidepressants – tricyclics decrease the phenytoin plasma concentration and the convulsive threshold

Antiepileptics – two or more antiepileptics enhance toxicity: monitoring of plasma concentrations required

Antiemetics – stemetil and derivatives lower convulsive threshold

Antihypertensives – nifedipine increases phenytoin plasma concentration; the effect of nifedipine is reduced

Anxiolytics and hypnotics – diazepam can increase or decrease plasma phenytoin concentration

Corticosteroids – metabolism is increased, therefore effect is decreased

Contraceptives – metabolism of oral contraceptives is increased, therefore their effect is decreased

Vitamins – the plasma phenytoin concentration is lowered by folic acid: vitamin D supplements may be required.

Phenobarbitone

Alcohol – increased sedative effect

Antibiotics – metabolism of metronidazole is increased, therefore the effect is decreased

Anticoagulants – metabolism of warfarin increased, therefore effect decreased

Antidepressants – tricyclics decrease the plasma concentration and the convulsive threshold

Antiepileptics – as for phenytoin, requires dose monitoring

Antiemetics – as for phenytoin

Antihypertensives – effect of nifedipine reduced
Corticosteroids – as for phenytoin
Contraceptives – as for phenytoin
Folic acid – phenobarbitone has antifolate effect

Sodium valproate

Analgesics – aspirin enhances effect
Antacids – cimetidine increases the plasma levels of valproate
Antibiotics – erythromycin increases plasma levels of valproate
Antiemetics – as for phenytoin
Antiepileptics – with two or more, close monitoring is required
Anticoagulants – increased anticoagulant effect – monitoring of PT time required
Cholestyramine – decreases the absorption of valproate
Zidovudine – antagonism of the metabolism of zidovudine, therefore increased toxicity

Carbamazepine

Alcohol – enhanced CNS effects
Antidepressants – tricyclics have an accelerated metabolism, therefore decreased effect – monitoring required
Antiepileptics – plasma concentration effected by concomitant use, therefore careful plasma monitoring required
Anticoagulants – decreased anticoagulant effect of warfarin
Cimetidine – inhibits the metabolism of carbamazepine, therefore increases plasma concentration
Corticosteroids – carbamazepine increases the metabolism of both β and dexamethasone
Dextropropoxyphene – increases the effect of carbamazepine
Erythromycin – increased plasma concentrations of carbamazepine

Nifedipine – decreased antiepileptic effect
OCP – decreased contraceptive effect
Tramadol – decreased effect of tramadol

References

Briggs GG, Freeman RK, Yaffe SJ. Drugs in pregnancy and lactation: a reference guide to fetal and neonatal risk, 3rd edn. Baltimore: Williams & Wilkins, 1990

British Medical Association and Royal Pharmaceutical Society of Great Britain. British national formulary. Number 43, March 2002. Bath: Bath Press, 2002

Hale T. Medications and mothers' milk, 9th edn. USA: Pharmasoft Publications, 2000

Hopkins SJ. Drugs and pharmacology for nurses, 13th edn. Edinburgh: Churchill Livingstone, 1999

Little BB. Medication during pregnancy. In: James DK, Steer PJ, Weiner CP, Gonik B, eds. High risk pregnancy: management options, 2nd edn. London: WB Saunders, 1999; 617–638

Pharmacodynamic properties of phenobarbital – Gardenal Sodium®, *http://www.adhb.govt.nz/newborn/drug*. Rhone-Poulenc Rorer data sheets – Gardenal®

SPC from the eMC, Epanutin®, ready mixed, parenteral, Parke Davis, updated on the eMC 24/08/01

SPC from the eMC, Epilim®, Sanofi Synthelabo, updated on the eMC 20/08/01

SPC from the eMC, Tegretol® Chewtabs 100 mg, 200 mg, Tegretol® tablets 100 mg, 200 mg, 400 mg, Cephalon, updated on the eMC 13/11/01

Stockley IH (ed) Drug interactions. London: Pharmaceutical Press, 1999

BP	SODIUM VALPROATE
Proprietary	Epilim® (Sanofi Synthelabo) sodium valproate (non-proprietary, see BNF for details)
Group	anticonvulsant
Uses/indications	all forms of epilepsy
Type of drug	POM
Presentation	tablets, solution, syrup, powder for reconstitution
Dosage	oral: 600 mg–2.5 g/day in two divided doses IV/IVI: same as oral but over 3–5 minutes
Route of admin	oral, IV/IVI
Contraindications	**pregnancy and breastfeeding**, hepatic or renal impairment, SLE
Side effects	gastrointestinal disturbances, nausea, ataxia, tremor, weight gain, hair loss, hepatic impairment, disturbed platelet function, pancreatitis; multiple therapy requires care
Interactions	see beginning of chapter
Pharmacodynamic properties	likely mode of action is potentiation of the inhibitory action of GABA, through action on the further synthesis or metabolism of GABA

table continues

Fetal risk	spina bifida, neonatal bleeding, hepatotoxicity, fetal growth deficiency, hyperbilirubinaemia, fetal distress, craniofacial defects, urogenital defects, hypospadias up to 50%, retarded psychomotor development, digital abnormalities
Breastfeeding	secreted in breast milk – in low doses appears safe; high doses – insufficient information to qualify as safe

BP	PHENYTOIN
Proprietary	Epanutin® (Parke Davis), phenytoin (non-proprietary, see BNF for details)
Group	anticonvulsant/antiepileptic
Uses/indications	epilepsy, fits – not absence seizures, treatment of eclampsia
Type of drug	POM Class 1
Presentation	capsules, tablets, suspension
Dosage	with or after food: 150–300 mg/day in 1–2 divided doses or as per protocol (plasma values need evaluation and observation) IV: phenytoin sodium in treatment of eclampsia as per protocol
Route of admin	oral, IV
Contraindications	**pregnancy and breastfeeding,** hepatic impairment, hypersensitivity, shock
Side effects	**OVERDOSE:** no known antidote – possibly removed from plasma by haemodialysis nausea, vomiting, headache, tremor, insomnia, prolonged usage – hirsutism, coarse facies, acne, gingival hyperplasia, confusion
Interactions	see beginning of chapter
Pharmacodynamic properties	appears to stabilize rather than raise seizure threshold, and to prevent the spread of seizure activity rather than abolish the primary focus of seizure discharge. The mechanism is not fully understood but may include:

table continues

	• a reduction in sodium conductance by enhancing its extrusion, thereby preventing potential seizure activity
	• enhancing the action of GABA inhibition and reducing excitatory synaptic transmission
	• presynaptic reduction of calcium entry and block release of neurotransmitters
Fetal risk	in trimesters 1 and 3 teratogen; maternal folic acid supplements should be given under medical supervision, increased risk of haemorrhage in the neonate: prophylaxis with vitamin K recommended
Breastfeeding	secreted in breast milk, some minor effects noted, mother and child should be monitored, manufacturer advises avoidance unless necessary

BP	PHENOBARBITONE
Proprietary	Gardenal Sodium® (Concord), phenobarbital (Martindale)
Group	antiepileptic – barbiturate
Uses/indications	epilepsy – not absence seizures
Type of drug	POM, CD
Presentation	tablets, elixir, ampoules
Dosage	oral: 50–200 mg q.d.s. to a max. 600 mg/day
	IM: 50–200 mg q.d.s. to a max. 600 mg/day (plasma monitoring is less useful as tolerance occurs)
Route of admin	oral, IM, IV injection
Contraindications	**pregnancy, breastfeeding,** impaired hepatic or renal function, respiratory depression
Side effects	tolerance develops, drowsiness, neural depression, allergic skin reactions, overdose
Interactions	see beginning of chapter
Pharmacodynamic properties	a barbiturate which is an effective anticonvulsant. It appears to elevate the seizure threshold and limit the spread of seizure activity. The mechanism is unknown but may involve an increase in the GABA synergic systems
Fetal risk	in trimesters 1 and 3, a teratogen, particularly neural tube defects, hypoprothrombinaemia and withdrawal in infants with maternal treatment late

table continues

	in pregnancy, concomitant administration with other antiepileptics has been linked to haemorrhagic disease of the newborn within the first 24 hrs of life, prophylaxis with vitamin K is recommended
Breastfeeding	avoid where possible, drowsiness in infant and other minor effects reported. Mother and baby need to be monitored

BP	CARBAMAZEPINE
Proprietary	Tegretol® (Cephalon), carbamazepine (non-proprietary, see BNF for details)
Group	anticonvulsant
Uses/indications	epilepsy, generalized seizures and partial seizures, not absence seizures or myoclonic seizures (trigeminal neuralgia)
Type of drug	POM
Presentation	tablets, suppositories, liquid, chewtabs
Dosage	oral: initially 100–200 mg once or twice/day, usually 0.8–1.2 g in evenly divided doses p.r.: when oral not available – 125 mg is considered equal to 100 mg orally – dependent on response – maximum of 1 g daily in evenly divided doses
Route of admin	oral, p.r.
Contraindications	**pregnancy, breastfeeding,** history of bone marrow depression, hepatic/renal impairment, blood hepatic or skin disorders, glaucoma, sensitivity to either carbamazepine or structurally similar drugs, use of tricyclic or MAOI drugs
Side effects	side effects are common and appear dose related, resolving spontaneously or after transient dose reduction gastrointestinal disturbances, drowsiness, headaches visual disturbances, rashes, blood disorders, including thrombocytopenia, hepatic/renal disorders

table continues

Interactions	see beginning of chapter
Pharmacodynamic properties	exact mechanism unknown, but thought to stabilize hyperexcited nerve membranes, inhibiting repetitive neuronal discharges and reducing excitatory impulses. It also reduces glutamate release and blockades sodium channels, thereby stabilizing neuronal membranes and action potential
Fetal risk	animal studies show an increase in mortality if taken during organogenesis; later administration caused growth retardation in rat fetuses – women who take carbamazepine should be counselled for risk and given antenatal screening, and the benefits of administration should be weighed against the risks. There is also a theoretical risk of HDN in the neonate, therefore prophylactic vitamin K is recommended
Breastfeeding	excreted but considered safe

Chapter 7

Antidepressants

These are substances that aim to restore the balance of neurotransmitter substances in the brain, a deficiency of which is thought to contribute to depression. They are usually monoamine oxidase inhibitors (MAOIs) or tricyclic antidepressants.

The student should be aware of:

- The clinical signs and progression of ante and postnatal depression (PND)
- The maternal and fetal sequelae of therapy
- The local availability of counselling and facilities for treatment
- The consequences for lack of either diagnosis or treatment of depression
- The research into PND and its relation to hypothyroidism in certain cases.

The author recommends that drugs in this group should be individually investigated, as psychiatry is a specialized field and most antidepressants require monitoring in pregnancy and breastfeeding.

References

Briggs GG, Freeman RK, Yaffe SJ. Drugs in pregnancy and lactation : a reference guide to fetal and neonatal risk, 3rd edn. Baltimore: Williams & Wilkins, 1990

British Medical Association and Royal Pharmaceutical Society of
    Great Britain. British national formulary. Number 43, March
    2002. Bath: Bath Press, 2002

Hale T. Medications and mothers' milk, 9th edn. USA: Pharmasoft
    Publications, 2000

Hopkins SJ. Drugs and pharmacology for nurses, 13th edn.
    Edinburgh: Churchill Livingstone, 1999

Little BB. Medication during pregnancy. In: James DK, Steer PJ,
    Weiner CP, Gonik B, eds. High risk pregnancy: management
    options, 2nd edn. London: WB Saunders, 1999; 617–638

SPC from the eMC, Prothiaden® tablets 75 mg, Abbott
    Laboratories Ltd, updated on the eMC 04/03/02

SPC from the eMC, Cyclogest®, Shire Pharmaceuticals Ltd,
    updated on the eMC 05/10/01

SPC from the eMC, Prozac®, Eli Lilley & Co.Ltd, updated on the
    eMC 17/08/01

Stockley IH (ed) Drug interactions. London: Pharmaceutical Press,
    1999

BP	DOTHIEPIN HYDROCHLORIDE (DOSULEPIN)
Proprietary	Prothiaden® (Abbot Laboratories Ltd)
Group	antidepressant – tricyclic
Uses/indications	depression where sedation is required, i.e. postnatal depression
Type of drug	POM
Presentation	capsules, tablets
Dosage	oral: 75 mg daily (divided or single) increased to 150–225 mg daily
Route of admin	oral
Contraindications	recent myocardial infarction, mania
Side effects	dry mouth, sedation, blurred vision, cardiovascular disturbances, blood sugar changes
Interactions	*alcohol* – avoid – enhanced sedative effect *antidepressants* – CNS excitation, hypertension with MAOIs – avoid for 2 weeks after stopping MAOI *antiepileptics* – convulsive threshold and tricyclic plasma concentration are lowered *antihistamines* – increased antimuscarinic and sedative effect, ventricular arrhythmias with terfenadine and astemizole *antihypertensives* – increases hypotensive effect *contraceptives* – antagonizes effect of antidepressants, but side effects increase the plasma concentration of tricyclics

table continues

Pharmacodynamic properties	tricyclic antidepressant that acts to increase transmitter levels at central synapses: this produces a clinical antidepressant effect. The inhibition of the re-uptake of noradrenaline (norepinephrine) and 5-hydoxytryptamine (5HT) and the uptake of dopamine produces adaptive changes in the brain which enhance the antidepressant effects
Fetal risk	tachycardia, irritability, muscle spasms and neonatal convulsions
Breastfeeding	amount secreted too small to be harmful in short-term use; accumulation may cause sedation and respiratory depression

BP	FLUOXETINE
Proprietary	Prozac® (Dista, Eli Lilley & Co. Ltd)
Group	antidepressant – SSRI
Uses/indications	depressive illness, bulimia nervosa, obsessive–compulsive disorder
Type of drug	POM
Presentation	capsules, liquid
Dosage	20 mg daily (varies according to condition)
Route of admin	oral
Contraindications	mania, cardiac disease, epilepsy, hepatic/renal impairment, pregnancy, breastfeeding, concomitant use of MAOI
Side effects	gastrointestinal disturbances, hypersensitivity, anxiety, palpitations, tremors, hair loss, confusion, hypotension, drowsiness, blood disorders, liver disturbances, suicidal thoughts
Interactions	*alcohol* – alcohol and SSRI are inadvisable *antidepressants* – enhance toxicity and levels require monitoring *antiepileptics* – carbamazepine and phenytoin enhance toxicity and levels require monitoring *anticoagulants* – warfarin – increased bleeding time, levels need monitoring *antihypertensives* – enhanced hypotensive effect
Pharmacodynamic properties	selective inhibitor of serotonin reuptake

table continues

Fetal risk	manufacturer advises use only if the benefits outweigh the risks
Breastfeeding	significant amounts are excreted into milk and considered moderately safe; manufacturer advises avoidance unless the benefits outweigh the risks

BP	PROGESTERONE
Proprietary	Cyclogest® (Hoechst)
Group	hormones – progesterone
Uses/indications	premenstrual syndrome, puerperal depression although there is no convincing evidence of physiological effectiveness, used for the alleviation of PND
Type of drug	POM
Presentation	suppositories
Dosage	200–400 mg
Route of admin	p.r., vaginally
Contraindications	diabetes, breastfeeding, hypertension, renal, hepatic or cardiac disease
Side effects	acne, urticaria, fluid retention, weight change, gastrointestinal disturbances, changes in libido
Interactions	none known
Pharmacodynamic properties	progestational steroid
Fetal risk	high doses can be teratogenic in the first trimester
Breastfeeding	high doses can inhibit or suppress lactation

Chapter 8

Antiemetics

These are drugs used to prevent or lessen nausea and vomiting. Some of these preparations may also be antipsychotics or antihistamines.

The student should be aware of:

- The actions of analgesics on the cerebral cortex
- The results of administration of the antipsychotic anti-emetics, i.e. their potentiating effects
- The appropriateness of treatment using anti-emetics, especially in early pregnancy.

References

Briggs GG, Freeman RK, Yaffe SJ. Drugs in pregnancy and lactation: a reference guide to fetal and neonatal risk, 3rd edn. Baltimore: Williams & Wilkins, 1990

British Medical Association and the Royal Pharmaceutical Society of Great Britain. British national formulary. Number 43, March 2002. Bath: Bath Press, 2002

Hale T. Medications and mothers' milk, 9th edn. USA: Pharmasoft Publications, 2000

Hopkins SJ. Drugs and pharmacology for nurses, 13th edn. Edinburgh: Churchill Livingstone, 1999

Little BB. Medication during pregnancy. In: James DK, Steer PJ, Weiner CP, Gonik B, eds. High risk pregnancy: management options, 2nd edn. London: WB Saunders, 1999; 617–638

SPC from the eMC, Largactil® injection, Hawgreen Ltd, updated on the eMC 29/08/01

SPC from the eMC, Valoid® 50 mg injection, CeNeS
    Pharmaceuticals, updated on the eMC 17/10/01
SPC from the eMC, Stemetil® injection, Castlemead Healthcare
    Ltd, updated on the eMC 23/08/01
SPC from the eMC, Maxolon® tablets 10 mg, Shire
    Pharmaceuticals Ltd, updated 23/07/01
Stockley IH (ed) Drug interactions. London: Pharmaceutical Press,
    1999
www.wholehealthmd.com/refshelf/drugs, the pharmacodynamic
    properties of chlorpromazine
www.edoc.co.za/medilink, the pharmacodynamic properties of
    promazine
Wyeth™ – data sheets – Sparine®

BP	PROCHLORPERAZINE
Proprietary	Stemetil® (Castlemead), Buccastem® (R and C), prochlorperazine (non-proprietary, see BNF)
Group	antiemetic – antipsychotic
Uses/indications	prophylaxis with the use of opioid analgesic, with excessive emesis
Type of drug	POM
Presentation	ampoules, tablets, suppositories
Dosage	IM: 12.5 mg 6–8-hrly oral: initially 20 mg then 10 mg after 2 hrs prevention of emesis: 5–10 mg b.d. or t.d.s. p.r.: 25 mg, followed if required by oral dose after 6 hrs migraine: 5 mg t.d.s.
Route of admin	IM, oral, p.r.
Contraindications	**pregnancy**, myasthenia gravis, cardiovascular and respiratory disease, epilepsy, phaeochromocytoma, liver or renal dysfunction, hypothyroidism
Side effects	*can cause prolonged labour and should be withheld until 3–4 cm dilation*, drowsiness, pallor, hypothermia, extrapyramidal effects, postural hypotension with tachycardia, liver dysfunction
Interactions	*alcohol* – increases the sedative effect particularly respiratory depression *antacids* – interfere with the absorption of oral Stemetil

table continues

	anaesthetics – increases their hypotensive effect *antiepileptics* – phenobarbitone – decreases plasma concentrations but is not thought to be clinically significant *antihistamines* – increased risk of ventricular arrhythmias with terfenadine *antihypertensives* – with methyldopa there is an increased risk of extrapyramidal effects
Pharmacodynamic properties	a potent phenothiazine neuroleptic used in nausea and vomiting, and in schizophrenia, acute mania and the management of anxiety
Fetal risk	in the first trimester there are reports of congenital defects associated with repeated use even at low doses, but single or occasional low doses appear safe, extrapyramidal symptoms in the neonate, lethargy and tremor, low APGARs, paradoxical hyperexcitability
Breastfeeding	amount probably too small to be excreted but avoid unless absolutely necessary; the manufacturer recommends against therapy during breastfeeding

BP	METOCLOPRAMIDE HYDROCHLORIDE
Proprietary	Maxolon® (Shire Pharmaceuticals Ltd)
Group	antiemetic
Uses/indications	nausea, vomiting
Type of drug	POM
Presentation	tablets, ampoules, infusion, oral suspension
Dosage	15–30 mg daily
Route of admin	IM, oral, IVI.
Contraindications	hepatic and renal impairment, may cause hypertension in phaeochromocytoma, caution in epilepsy
Side effects	extrapyramidal effects, hyperprolactinaemia
Interactions	*analgesics* – increases the absorption of aspirin and paracetamol, thereby enhancing their effect *opioid analgesics* – antagonize the effect on gastrointestinal activity.
Pharmacodynamic properties	action of metoclopramide is closely associated with the parasympathetic nervous control of the upper gastro-intestinal (GI) tract. It encourages normal peristaltic action and is indicated in conditions where disturbed GI motility is an underlying factor
Fetal risk	use with caution, there is no information on the long-term evaluation of infants exposed in utero
Breastfeeding	use with caution as there is a theoretical risk of potent central nervous system effects

BP	PROMAZINE HYDROCHLORIDE
Proprietary	Sparine® (Wyeth), promazine (non-proprietary, see BNF)
Group	antiemetic – antipsychotic
Uses/indications	relaxant, antiemetic in conjunction with opioids
Type of drug	POM
Presentation	ampoules, tablets, solution, suspension
Dosage	IM: 50 mg 6–8 hrly oral: 100–200 mg q.d.s.
Route of admin	IM, oral
Contraindications	as for prochlorperazine
Side effects	drowsiness, amnesia, pallor, extrapyramidal symptoms
Interactions	nil specific *phenothiazines*: *antacids* – reduce the absorption of phenothiazines *antidepressants* – tricyclics – increased antimuscarinic effects *antihypertensives* – hydrallazine enhances hypotensive effect *antipsychotics:* *alcohol* – enhanced sedative effect *anaesthetics* – enhanced hypotensive effect *analgesics* – opioids – enhanced hypotensive and sedative effects *antacids* – cimetidine – possibly enhances antipsychotic effects

table continues

	antihypertensives – enhanced hypotensive effect, increased risk of extrapyramidal effects *antidepressants* – tricyclics – increased plasma absorption and a possible increased risk of ventricular arrhythmias *antiemetics* – metoclopramide – increased risk of extrapyramidal effects *antiepileptics* – antagonism of the anticonvulsant effect *anxiolytics and hypnotics* – enhanced sedative effects
Pharmacodynamic properties	as for chlorpromazine
Fetal risk	consensus of research reports no adverse effects but use with caution because of potential teratogenicity and central nervous system effects on the neonate
Breastfeeding	as for prochlorperazine, but the manufacturer recommends that the product should not be used in conjunction with breastfeeding

BP	CHLORPROMAZINE
Proprietary	Largactil® (Rhone-Poulenc Rorer), chlorpromazine (non-proprietary, see BNF for details)
Group	antiemetic – antipsychotic, phenothiazine – neuroleptic
Uses/indications	nausea and vomiting
Type of drug	POM
Presentation	ampoules, tablets, suspension, suppositories (see below)
Dosage	IM: 25 mg then 25–50 mg 3–4-hrly until effective oral: 10–25 mg 4–6-hrly p.r.: 100 mg 6–8-hrly (unlicensed)
Route of admin	IM, oral, (p.r.)
Contraindications	phaeochromocytoma, epilepsy, myasthenia gravis, hepatic or renal dysfunction, hypothyroidism
Side effects	as for prochlorperazine
Interactions	the action of this drug is intensified by alcohol, other neuroleptics, barbiturates and sedatives, with respiratory depression a particular side effect *anticholinergics* – enhance the antipsychotic effect *antiepileptics* – interferes with the plasma concentrations of drugs but is not clinically significant otherwise as for prochlorperazine

table continues

Pharmacodynamic properties	inhibits the activity of the brain chemical dopamine. This prevents the overstimulation of specific nerve centres which may be responsible for certain psychiatric disorders, and also suppresses the trigger zones of the brain that control hiccuping and vomiting
Fetal risk	as for prochlorperazine
Breastfeeding	as for prochlorperazine

BP	CYCLIZINE
Proprietary	Valoid® (CeNeS Pharmaceuticals)
Group	anticholinergic – antiemetic
Uses/indications	prevention and treatment of nausea and vomiting
Type of drug	POM
Presentation	ampoules
Dosage	IM or IV: 50 mg can be t.d.s.
	Postop: slow IV injection 20 minutes before the end of surgery
Route of admin	IM, IV
Contraindications	hypersensitivity to cyclizine, cardiac disease
Side effects	hypotension, fall in cardiac output, urticaria, rash, drowsiness, oropharyngeal dryness, tachycardia, blurred vision, urinary retention, constipation
Interactions	*alcohol* – enhances the effect of cyclizine
	analgesics – enhances the soporific effect of pethidine
	anticholinergics – concomitant use gives enhanced effects
	*CNS suppressant*s – enhances the effect of cyclizine
Pharmacodynamic properties	a histamine H_1 receptor antagonist, cyclizine has a low incidence of drowsiness but has antiemetic and anticholinergic properties. The exact mechanism is unknown, but it is thought

table continues

	to act to increase lower oesophageal sphincter tone, and it may also have an inhibitory effect on the emetic centre located in the midbrain
Fetal risk	manufacturer advises that animal studies indicate teratogenicity
Breastfeeding	no data available from controlled studies in breastfeeding women, but considered moderately safe

Chapter 9

Antihypertensives

These are substances used to control or modify blood pressure, either by reducing peripheral resistance or blocking α or β adrenoreceptors in the heart, or by reducing the central flow of impulses to the sympathetic nerves and decreasing the release of noradrenaline (norepinephrine) at adrenergic nerve endings.

The student should be aware of:

- The physiology and pathophysiology of blood pressure
- The aetiology, pathophysiology and progression of pregnancy-induced hypertension and pre-eclampsia
- The difference between essential hypertension and pregnancy-induced hypertension and pre-eclampsia/eclampsia
- The maternal and fetal sequelae of therapy using these substances
- The local protocols for treatment in cases of eclampsia (see emergency drugs).

References

Briggs GG, Freeman RK, Yaffe SJ. Drugs in pregnancy and lactation: a reference guide to fetal and neonatal risk, 3rd edn. Baltimore: Williams & Wilkins, 1990

British Medical Association and the Royal Pharmaceutical Society of Great Britain. British national formulary. Number 43, March 2002. Bath: Bath Press, 2002

Hale T. Medications and mothers' milk, 9th edn. USA: Pharmasoft Publications, 2000

Hallak M. Hypertension in pregnancy. In: James DK, Steer PJ, Weiner CP, Gonik B (eds) High risk pregnancy: management options, 2nd edn. London: WB Saunders, 1999; 639–663

Hopkins SJ. Drugs and pharmacology for nurses, 13th edn. Edinburgh: Churchill Livingstone, 1999

Little BB. Medication during pregnancy. In: James DK, Steer PJ, Weiner CP, Gonik B (eds) High risk pregnancy: management options, 2nd edn. London: WB Saunders, 1999; 617–638

Lloyd C, Lewis VM. Hypertensive disorders of pregnancy. In: Bennett VR, Brown LK (eds) Myles textbook for midwives, 13th edn. Edinburgh: Churchill Livingstone, 1999; 315–328

Royal College of Obstetricians and Gynaecologists. Management of eclampsia. Clinical Greentop Guidelines No.10. July 1999, reviewed July 2002

SPC from the eMC, Trandate® 100 mg, Celltech, updated from the eMC 20/06/01

SPC from the eMC, Adalat®, Bayer PLC, updated on the eMC 16/08/01

SPC from the eMC, Aldomet® 250 mg and 500 mg tablets, Merck Sharp and Dohme Ltd, updated from the eMC 16/08/01

Stockley IH (ed) Drug interactions. London: Pharmaceutical Press, 1999

http://www.wholehealthmd.com/refshelf/drugs – pharmacodynamic properties of nifedipine and methyldopa

BP	NIFEDIPINE
Proprietary	Adalat® (Bayer), nifedipine (non-proprietary, see BNF)
Group	calcium channel blocker, hypotensive, vasodilator
Uses/indications	hypertensive crisis, uncontrolled hypertension
Type of drug	POM
Presentation	capsules, tablets (slow release)
Dosage	10 mg stat, 10 mg b.d.
Route of admin	oral (preferably sublingual during hypertensive crisis)
Contraindications	continuous use in pregnancy, breastfeeding, hypersensitivity
Side effects.	headache, flushing, dizziness, oedema, headache, may inhibit labour **CAUTION:** stop treatment if ischaemic pain occurs within 30–60 minutes of administration; treatment with short-acting nifedipine, i.e. during a crisis, can induce an exaggerated fall in blood pressure and reflex tachycardia, which may cause complications such as cerebrovascular accident/ischaemia or myocardial ischaemia **EXTREME CAUTION** when using magnesium sulphate
Interactions	do not take with grapefruit juice *antihypertensives* – causes severe hypotension and possible heart failure

table continues

	cimetidine – potentiates the hypotensive effect as metabolism of nifedipine is inhibited *phenytoin* – concomitant administration can reduce the effect of nifedipine – monitor plasma levels of anticonvulsants *erythromycin* – may potentiate nifedipine effects *insulin* – possible impaired glucose tolerance
Pharmacodynamic properties	selective calcium channel blocker with mostly vascular effects. It is a specific and potent calcium antagonist which relaxes smooth arterial muscle, causing arteries to widen, thereby reducing the resistance in coronary and peripheral circulation. This reduces blood pressure and decreases the heart's overall workload
Fetal risk	toxicity in animals, hypotensive effect can reduce placental flow and cause decrease in fetal oxygenation, may inhibit labour
Breastfeeding	considered safe 3–4 hrs after dose, but manufacturer advises avoidance

BP	METHYLDOPA
Proprietary	methyldopa (non-proprietary see BNF), Aldomet® (MSD)
Group	centrally acting antihypertensive
Uses/indications	hypertension in pregnancy, hypertensive crisis where immediate effect is not necessary, can be used by asthmatics
Type of drug	POM
Presentation	tablets, suspension, ampoules
Dosage	oral: 250 mg b.d. (t.d.s.) max. 3 g/day, gradually increased at intervals of 2 days or more IVI: 250–500 mg q.d.s.
Route of admin	oral, IVI
Contraindications	history of depression, liver disease, phaeochromocytoma, concurrent treatment with MAOIs, porphyria, history of hepatic or renal dysfunction
Side effects	reduced if under 1 g/day, dry mouth, sedation, depression, fluid retention, haemolytic anaemia, SLE-like syndrome, postural hypotension, gastrointestinal disturbances, dizziness, headache, numbness, hyperprolactinaemia, nightmares, mild psychosis, blood disorders, nasal congestion, nerve and joint pain, hepatic disorders, may interfere with laboratory results – 20% have a positive DCT – advise laboratory of treatment if requiring crossmatch

table continues

Interactions	effect is diminished by *sympathomimetics*, *phenothiazines*, *tricyclic antidepressants and MAOIs* *alcohol* – enhances hypotensive effect *anaesthetics* – enhances hypotensive effect ++ *analgesics* – NSAIDs enhance hypotensive effect *antihypertensives* – potentiates hypotensive effect *anxiolytics and hypnotics* – enhance hypotensive effect *corticosteroids* – antagonize hypotensive effect *contraceptives* – antagonize hypotensive effect *iron* – possible reduction in the bioavailability of ferrous sulphate or ferrous gluconate if ingested with methyldopa *salbutamol* – use with caution as it can potentiate the hypotensive effect
Pharmacodynamic properties	acts on certain areas in the CNS that regulate heart activity and the smooth muscle surrounding the arteries: the vessels widen and relax, which in turn reduces blood pressure. Withdrawal of the drug is followed by a return of hypertension within 48 hrs
Fetal risk	crosses the placental barrier and is present in cord blood, but there are no reports of fetal or neonatal abnormalities although there is a theoretical risk of toxicity/ teratogenicity with multiple therapy

table continues

Breastfeeding	found in breast milk, and although there are no obvious effects the manufacturer advises that lactating mothers be warned of its presence and possible risk, but does not advise avoidance

BP	HYDRALLAZINE HYDROCHLORIDE
Proprietary	Hydrallazine (non-proprietary see BNF), Apresoline® (Alliance)
Group	antihypertensive – vasodilator
Uses/indications	raised diastolic blood pressure used concomitantly with other therapies, i.e. beta-blockers or during a hypertensive crisis
Type of drug	POM
Presentation	tablets, injection, powder for reconstitution
Dosage	oral: 25–50 mg b.d.
	IV injection: 5–10 mg over 20 minutes, repeated after 20–30 minutes – diluted with NaCl 0.9%
	IV infusion: 200–300 µg/min
	maintenance: 5–150 µg/min
Route of admin	oral, IV injection or infusion
Contraindications	systemic lupus erythematosus (SLE), tachycardia, hepatic, renal or cardiac dysfunction or cerebrovascular accident
Side effects.	nausea, postural hypotension, tachycardia, palpitations, flushing, fluid retention, after prolonged or high-dose therapy SLE-like syndrome, headache, dizziness, joint muscle and nerve pain, nasal congestion, blood disorders, liver and renal disorders
Interactions	*alcohol* – enhances hypotensive effect *anaesthetics* – enhances hypotensive effect

table continues

	analgesics – NSAIDs enhance hypotensive effect *antihypertensives* – enhance hypotensive effect *anxiolytics and hypnotics* – enhance the hypotensive effects *contraceptives* – combined oral contraceptives antagonize the hypotensive effect
Pharmacodynamic properties	acts on the smooth muscle tissue surrounding the arteries, causing them to relax and hence the blood pressure to fall
Fetal risk	toxicity in animals, therefore considered a teratogen, although there are no reported links to congenital defects in humans. Avoid before the third trimester, but there are no reports of serious harm
Breastfeeding	considered safe but monitor infant

BP	LABETALOL HYDROCHLORIDE
Proprietary	Labetalol (non-proprietary see BNF), Trandate® (Celltech)
Group	antihypertensive – α and β adrenoreceptor blocker
Uses/indications	hypertension in pregnancy, hypertensive crisis
Type of drug	POM
Presentation	tablets, ampoules
Dosage	oral: initial dose 100 mg b.d. increased at weekly intervals by 100 mg b.d., i.e. to 200 mg b.d.
	in the 2nd and 3rd trimesters further dose titration to t.d.s., ranging 100–400 mg t.d.s.
	can be increased up to 800 mg in three to four evenly divided doses/day (max. 2.4 g daily)
	IV injection: 50 mg over 1 minute repeated after 5 minutes (max. 200 mg)
	IV infusion: 20 mg/hr doubled after 30 minutes (max. 160 mg/hr)
Route of admin	oral, IV injection or infusion
Contraindications	asthma, chronic obstructive airways disease, wheezing, phaeochromocytoma, bradycardia, sensitivity to labetalol, heart block, Raynaud's disease, with caution in patients with psoriasis
Side effects	postural hypotension – particularly 3 hrs after IV administration, tiredness, weakness, epigastric pain, difficulty with

table continues

	micturition, scalp tingling, tremor in pregnant patients
Interactions	*alcohol* – enhances hypotensives effect as delays metabolism of labetalol *anaesthetics* – enhance hypotensive effect *analgesics* – NSAIDs enhance hypotensive effects *antacids* – cimetidine inhibits the metabolism and therefore increases the plasma concentration of labetalol *antidepressants* – tricyclics cause tremor, MAOIs not recommended *antidiabetics* – enhanced hypoglycaemic effects and masks warning signs such as tremor *antihistamines* – increased risk of ventricular arrhythmia with terfenadine *antihypertensives* – concomitant use may cause severe hypotension *anxiolytics and hypnotics* – enhance the hypotensive effect *corticosteroids* – antagonize the hypotensive effect *ergometrine* – increases peripheral vasoconstriction *contraceptives* – combined oral contraceptives antagonize the hypotensive effect
Pharmacodynamic properties	works by blocking peripheral arteriolar α receptors and this reduces peripheral resistance. A concurrent β-blockade protects the heart from any reflux effects. Cardiac output is not significantly reduced at rest or after moderate exercise, i.e. the

table continues

	increase in systolic pressure during exercise is reduced and the diastolic pressure remains essentially normal
Fetal risk	caution in use – β blockers reduce placental perfusion, leading to a risk of intrauterine death, premature delivery, fetal growth deficiency, and increased risk of neonatal hypoglycaemia and bradycardia, respiratory depression and neonatal jaundice. The risk is greater in severe hypertension and with multiple therapy, although these effects may be due to the disease itself and not the therapy. Symptoms can develop 1–2 days post delivery
Breastfeeding	considered safe but monitor infant carefully

Chapter 10

Antiseptics

These substances are also known as disinfectants, bacteriostats, bactericides and germicides. They will inhibit the growth of or kill micro-organisms. Antiseptics are usually applied to the body and disinfectants to equipment etc. Skin cleansers are also included in this chapter.

The student should be aware of:

- The difference between antiseptics and antibiotics.

References

British Medical Association and Royal Pharmaceutical Society of Great Britain. British national formulary. Number 43, March 2002. Bath: Bath Press, 2002

Hale T. Medications and mothers' milk, 9th edn. USA: Pharmasoft Publications, 2000

Hopkins SJ. Drugs and pharmacology for nurses, 13th edn. Edinburgh: Churchill Livingstone, 1999

SPC from the eMC, Hibiscrub®, SSL International Ltd, updated on the eMC 10/08/01

SPC from the eMC, Hibitane® Obstetric Cream, Bioglan Laboratories Ltd, updated on the eMC 31/08/98

SPC from the eMC, Betadine® Sugical Scrub, SSL International Ltd, updated on the eMC 03/07/01

SPC from the eMC, Mediswabs-H®, SSL International Ltd, updated on the eMC 03/07/01

SPC from the eMC, Sterets®, SSL International Ltd, updated 03/07/01

BP	SURGICAL ALCOHOL (ISOPROPYL ALCOHOL)
Proprietary	Mediswab® (SSL International), Sterets® (SSL International)
Group	alcohol-based cleanser
Uses/indications	preparation of the skin prior to injection
Type of drug	GSL
Presentation	liquid, injection swabs
Dosage	N/A
Route of admin	topical
Contraindications	broken skin, patients with burns, prior to using diathermy
Side effects	
Interactions	N/A
Pharmacodynamic properties	70% isopropyl alcohol has disinfectant properties and when used in combination with chlorhexidine has antimicrobial qualities, therefore it is used to clean the skin and reduce the bacteriological count prior to injection or surgery
Fetal risk	N/A
Breastfeeding	N/A

BP	SODIUM CHLORIDE
Proprietary	Normasol® (SSL International), sodium chloride (non-proprietary see BNF)
Group	saline skin cleanser
Uses/indications	cleansing of skin and wounds
Type of drug	
Presentation	sterile solution in ampoules and sachets
Dosage	N/A
Route of admin	topical
Contraindications	N/A
Side effects	N/A
Interactions	N/A
Fetal risk	N/A
Breastfeeding	N/A

BP	POVIDONE–IODINE
Proprietary	Betadine® (SSL International), Savlon® powder-spray (Novartis Consumer Health)
Group	antiseptic – iodine compounds
Uses/indications	skin disinfection, pre- and postoperative, caution with diathermy
Type of drug	N/A
Presentation	prepared solutions, powders
Dosage	N/A
Route of admin	topical
Contraindications	iodine sensitivity, renal impairment, regular use in patients or users with thyroid disorders
Side effects	sensitivity
Interactions	N/A
Pharmacodynamic properties	the povidone–iodine slowly liberates iodine on contact with the skin and mucous membranes and acts as a microbicide, effectively 'suffocating' the microbe by displacing its oxygen supply and altering the stability of the microbial cell membrane
Fetal risk	avoid use on very low-birthweight babies, avoid regular use in pregnancy and lactation, as iodine compounds cross the placenta and are secreted in breast milk

table continues

| Breastfeeding | secreted in breast milk, and although no adverse effects have been reported it should be considered hazardous and the possible benefits should be weighed against the risks of fetal thyroid dysfunction and maldevelopment |

BP	CHLORHEXIDINE
Proprietary	Hibiscrub® (SSL International), Hibisol® (SSL International), Hibitane® (Bioglan), Chlorhexidine® (non-proprietary see BNF)
Group	antiseptic – chlorhexidine salts, phenyl derivative
Uses/indications	skin preparation prior to surgery, cleansing of perineum and vulva, lubrication of the midwife's hands
Type of drug	N/A
Presentation	prepared solutions of varying concentrations
Dosage	N/A
Route of admin	topical
Contraindications	hypersensitivity, avoid contact with the eyes, brain meninges and middle ear, not suitable before diathermy
Side effects	sensitivity
Interactions	N/A
Pharmacodynamic properties	wide range of antimicrobial activities against Gram-positive and -negative vegetative bacteria, dermatologic fungi and lipophilic viruses. It is inactive against bacterial spores except at elevated temperatures. Its cationic nature means that it binds strongly to skin, mucosa and other tissues and is very poorly absorbed, therefore there are no detectable levels after oral or skin contact
Fetal risk	N/A
Breastfeeding	considered safe

BP	CHLORHEXIDINE CETRIMIDE SOLUTION
Proprietary	Savlon®
Group	antiseptic – phenyl derivative
Uses/indications	general-purpose antiseptic, disinfectant and detergent
Type of drug	GSL
Presentation	liquid – chlorhexidine 1.5%:cetrimide 15 %
Dosage	as instructed
Route of admin	topical
Contraindications	sensitivity
Side effects	contamination by *Pseudomonas aeruginosa* – store as sterile solutions in screwtop bottles
Interactions	N/A
Fetal risk	N/A
Breastfeeding	N/A

Chapter 11

Contraceptives

This is a general term to describe an agent used to prevent conception. Those mentioned in this chapter are hormonal therapies and not devices.

The student should be aware of:

- Clause 3 of the Definition of a midwife: 'the midwife has an important task in health counselling and education. . . . which extends to family planning' (Midwives' Code of Practice,1998)
- The availability of contraception
- The importance of family planning
- The process of contraception with a view to usage of emergency contraception
- The appropriateness of the contraceptive prescribed
- The importance of counselling – advice on bleeding, missed pills, diarrhoea and vomiting, antibiotic administration, and cessation of oral contraception prior to surgery.

References

Briggs GG, Freeman RK, Yaffe SJ. Drugs in pregnancy and lactation: a reference guide to fetal and neonatal risk, 3rd edn. Baltimore: Williams & Wilkins, 1990

British Medical Association and the Royal Pharmaceutical Society of Great Britain. British national formulary. Number 43, March 2002. Bath: Bath Press, 2002

Hale T. Medications and mothers' milk, 9th edn. USA: Pharmasoft Publications, 2000

Hopkins SJ. Drugs and pharmacology for nurses, 13th edn. Edinburgh: Churchill Livingstone, 1999

Little BB. Medication during pregnancy: In James DK, Steer PJ, Weiner CP, Gonik B (eds) High risk pregnancy: management options, 2nd edn. London: WB Saunders, 1999; 617–638

SPC from the eMC, Femodene®, Schering Healthcare Ltd, updated on the eMC 08/01/02

SPC from the eMC, Microgynon 30®, Schering Healthcare Ltd, updated on the eMC 29/06/00

SPC from the eMC, Eugynon 30®, Schering Healthcare Ltd, updated on the eMC 18/01/02

SPC from the eMC, Minulet®, Wyeth Laboratories updated on the eMC 14/08/00

SPC from the eMC, Micronor®, Janssen Cilag Ltd, updated on the eMC 22/08/01

SPC from the eMC, Microval®, Wyeth Laboratories, updated on the eMC 24/08/01

SPC from the eMC, Norgeston®, Schering Healthcare Limited, updated on the eMC 18/07/01

SPC from the eMC, Neogest®, Schering Healthcare Ltd, revised on the eMC April 2000

SPC from the eMC, Femulen®, Pharmacia, updated on the eMC 23/08/01

SPC from the eMC, Depoprovera®, Pharmacia, updated on the eMC 25/10/01

SPC from the eMC, Noristerat ®, Schering Healthcare Ltd, revised on the eMC 18/01/96

SPC from the eMC, Levonelle–2®, Schering Healthcare Ltd, revised on the eMC 19/10/01

SPC from the eMC, Implanon®, Organon Laboratories Ltd, updated on the eMC 30/05/02

Stockley IH (ed) Drug interactions. London: Pharmaceutical Press, 1999

UKCC. Midwives' rules and code of practice. London: UKCC, 1998

Further Reading

Keller S. When to begin postpartum methods. Network 1995:15:18–23

BP	LEVONORGESTREL
Proprietary	Levonelle-2® (Schering Health)
Group	contraceptive – emergency
Uses/indications	emergency contraception within 3 days (72 hrs) of unprotected intercourse
Type of drug	POM (GSL over 16 yrs of age by pharmacists only)
Presentation	tablets
Dosage	initial dose 750 µg followed (12 hrs but no later than 16 hrs) by second dose of 750 µg
Route of admin	oral
Contraindications	**pregnancy,** porphyria, overdue menstrual bleeding or unprotected intercourse more than 72 hrs previously
Side effects	nausea, abdominal pain, vomiting, headache, fatigue, breast discomfort
Interactions	The effectiveness of this drug is *reduced* by *enzyme-inducing drugs,* in which case increase the initial dose to 1.5 mg followed in 12 hrs by 750 µg. These include antiepileptics, St John's Wort, rifamycin family of antibiotics
Pharmacodynamic properties	inhibits ovulation if taken in the preovulatory stage, and also causes endometrial changes which discourage implantation. However, once implantation has occurred then it is no longer an

table continues

	effective contraceptive. It is effective up to 85% if given within 72 hrs of intercourse (95% within 24 hrs, 85% within 24–48 hrs, 58% within 48–72 hrs)
Fetal risk	**abortifacient,** but pregnancy may continue, monitor for signs of ectopic pregnancy. In theory, because there is no organogenesis at 72 hrs there should be no teratogenicity
Breastfeeding	exposure of the infant is reduced if the mother avoids nursing post medication

BP	ETONOGESTREL
Proprietary	Implanon® (Organon)
Group	parenteral progesterone-only contraceptive
Uses/indications	contraception effective for 3 yrs – rapidly reversible on removal
Type of drug	POM
Presentation	flexible rod
Dosage	68 mg of etonogestrel in each rod with no previous hormonal contraception: one implant in the first 5 days of the cycle parturition/abortion in 2nd trimester: one implant 21–28 days after delivery or abortion
Route of admin	subdermal
Contraindications	as for progesterone-only pill
Side effects	aching, pain at site, tiredness, acne, alopecia, headache, dizziness, depression, mood swings, libido changes, gastrointestinal disturbances, weight changes, menstrual symptoms, occasional hypertension, increased risk of DVT
Interactions	as for progesterone-only pill
Pharmacodynamic properties	a progestagen that inhibits progesterone receptors in target organs. Primarily it works to inhibit ovulation, and also to thicken the cervical mucus, making it hostile to spermatozoa
Fetal risk	as for progesterone-only pill
Breastfeeding	as for progesterone-only pill

BP	MEDROXYPROGESTERONE ACETATE
Proprietary	Depoprovera® (Pharmacia)
Group	parenteral progesterone-only contraceptive
Uses/indications	interim or long-term contraception – 12 weeks' duration in long-term use reduce the term to 10 weeks
Type of drug	POM
Presentation	aqueous suspension in vials
Dosage	150 mg in first 5 days of menstrual cycle or within 5 days of parturition; repeat in 12 weeks
Route of admin	IM
Contraindications	as for oral preparations
Side effects	all-over rash, nausea, giddiness, heavy bleeding during menses or postpartum, delay in return of fertility, menstrual disturbances
Interactions	as for oral preparations
Pharmacodynamic properties	exerts an anti-androgenic and anti-gonadotrophic effect which inhibits ovulation and endometrial preparation for pregnancy
Fetal risk	possible increase in low birthweight that is associated with increased risk of neonatal death – although the attributable risk is low as pregnancies are uncommon. Those exposed show no adverse effects
Breastfeeding	withhold first dose until 5–6 weeks postpartum – but preparation does not suppress lactation

BP	NORETHISTERONE ENANTHATE
Proprietary	Noristerat® (Schering Health)
Group	parenteral progesterone-only contraceptive
Uses/indications	short-term or interim contraception, 8 weeks' duration
Type of drug	POM
Presentation	oily preparation in ampoules
Dosage	deep IM: 200 mg in first 5 days of cycle or immediately following parturition, repeat in 8 weeks
Route of admin	deep IM
Contraindications	as for oral preparations
Side effects	as for oral preparations
Interactions	as for oral preparations
Fetal risk	as for oral preparations
Breastfeeding	withhold when neonate has severe jaundice requiring medical treatment may also suppress lactation in high doses and alter its composition, therefore use the lowest effective dose

BP	PROGESTERONE-ONLY PILL (POP)
Proprietary	Micronor® (Janssen-Cilag), Femulen® (Pharmacia), Microval® (Wyeth), Norgeston® (Schering Health), Neogest® (Pharmacia), Noriday® (Pharmacia)
Group	contraceptive – hormonal
Uses/indications	contraception, alternative to oestrogens – higher failure rate, suitable in smokers, hypertension, valvular heart disease, diabetes mellitus, migraine, predisposition to or history of thrombosis or venous thrombosis
Type of drug	POM
Presentation	tablets in cyclical packs
Dosage	usually one tablet/day, but refer to pack instructions – must be taken at the same time each day
	postpartum – commence after 3 weeks – breakthrough bleeding if earlier – mothers should also be aware of the increased risk of thromboembolic disorders
Route of admin	oral
Contraindications	pregnancy, undiagnosed vaginal bleeding, severe arterial disease, existing thrombophlebitis or thromboembolic disorders, cerebrovascular disease, porphyria, heart disease including myocardial infarction, malabsorption syndromes, liver disease, sex steroid-dependent cancers, past ectopic pregnancy, functional ovarian cysts,

table continues

	cholestatic jaundice, pruritus of pregnancy, Dubin–Johnson syndrome, Rotor syndrome, history of herpes gestationis, disorders of lipid metabolism
Side effects	menstrual irregularities, nausea, vomiting, menstrual symptoms, weight change, depression, dizziness, loss of libido, headaches, chloasma
Interactions	*antibiotics* – rifamycins – increase metabolism and therefore reduce effect *anticoagulants* – antagonizes effect of warfarin *antidiabetics* – antagonizes the hypoglycaemic effects *antiepileptics* – reduce contraceptive effect *St John's Wort* – can lead to potential loss of contraceptive effect
Pharmacodynamic properties	POPs have a progestational effect on the endometrium and cervical mucus that discourages implantation and decreases corpus luteum function
Fetal risk	high doses may be teratogenic in the first trimester (US studies have found a 0.07 % risk) masculinization of the fetus, although only with very high progesterone doses
Breastfeeding	not contraindicated, but not before 3 weeks postpartum. Manufacturer advises avoidance, as small amounts of active ingredients are excreted in breast milk and the effects on the infant are unknown

BP	COMBINED OESTROGEN/PROGESTOGEN ORAL CONTRACEPTIVE (COC)
Proprietary	various – Femodene® (Schering Health), Microgynon 30® (Schering Health), Eugynon 30® (Schering Health), Minulet® (Wyeth) etc
Group	contraceptive – hormonal
Uses/indications	contraception, menstrual symptoms
Type of drug	POM
Presentation	tablets in packs for 1 month, with days numbered
Dosage	usually one tablet/day, but refer to pack for instructions *postpartum* (not breastfeeding) – commence at 3 weeks postpartum – there is an increased risk of DVT if commenced earlier – patient must be fully ambulant, with no puerperal complications and be counselled for the risk of DVT *breastfeeding* – not recommended until weaning or at least 6 months if unable to obtain other contraception *miscarriage or abortion* – commence same day if possible
Route of admin	oral

table continues

Contraindications	pregnancy, migraine, liver disease including cholestatic jaundice, history of pruritus in pregnancy, breastfeeding, prothrombotic coagulation disorders, previous history or strong familial history of DVT, undiagnosed vaginal bleeding, breast or genital tract carcinoma
	CAUTION: arterial disease, smoking, hypertension, obesity, diabetes mellitus with retinopathy and nephropathy, ischaemic heart disease, varicosities, depression, inflammatory bowel disease, Rotor syndrome, Dubin–Johnson syndrome, sickle cell anaemia, history of herpes gestationis, disorders of lipid metabolism. Stop prior to major surgery or surgery to the legs, or with long-term immobilization – do not stop for minor surgery with short anaesthetic duration, e.g. laparoscopy or tooth extraction
Side effects	nausea, vomiting, headache, breast tenderness, changes in body weight, libido changes, DVT, intra-cyclic bleeding, amenorrhoea, decreased menstrual bleeding, depression, impaired liver function
Interactions	*antibiotics* – broad spectrum – reduce effect *anticoagulants* – antagonizes the effect of warfarin

table continues

	antidepressants – tricyclics – antagonizes the antidepressant effects but increases the side effects because of the increased plasma concentration of tricyclics
	antidiabetics – antagonism of the hypoglycaemic effect
	antiepileptics – carbamazepine, phenobarbital, phenytoin accelerate metabolism and reduce contraceptive effect
	antihypertensives – antagonize hypotensive effect
Pharmacodynamic properties	the combination of these preparations acts to inhibit ovulation by suppressing the mid-cycle surge of luteinizing hormone, thickening the cervical mucus as a barrier to sperm and rendering the endometrium unresponsive to implantation
Fetal risk	evidence suggests no harmful effects to fetus, although there is teratogenicity in animals (US studies have found a small risk of 0.07% of all pregnancies exposed to the oral contraceptive pill)
Breastfeeding	suppressed lactation, contraindicated until at least 6 months after birth

Chapter 12

Antihistamines

Histamine is present in animal tissues and some release occurs after injury, but also after an allergic reaction, and gives rise to urticaria, asthma, hayfever and ultimately **anaphylaxis**.

Antihistamines are palliative agents because they neither destroy nor prevent the release of histamine, but act by blocking access to histamine receptor sites and thereby inhibit an allergic reaction.

Antihistamines are usually thought of as being taken orally, but they can be injected, for example chlorpheniramine and promazine are used as adjuncts to adrenaline (epinephrine) in the treatment of anaphylaxis. Antihistamines are used in the treatment of nausea and vomiting, and for the purposes of this book are listed in Chapter 8 – Antiemetics.

The student should be aware of:

- The physiology related to allergic response
- The most common factors causing allergic response
- Treatment for anaphylactic shock
- Interactions of drug therapy that may produce an allergic response, e.g. with cimetidine.

References

Briggs GG, Freeman RK, Yaffe SJ. Drugs in pregnancy and lactation: a reference guide to fetal and neonatal risk, 3rd edn. Baltimore: Williams & Wilkins, 1990

British Medical Association and the Royal Pharmaceutical Society of Great Britain. British national formulary. Number 43, March 2002. Bath: Bath Press, 2002

Hale T. Medications and mothers' milk, 9th edn. USA: Pharmasoft Publications, 2000

Hopkins SJ. Drugs and pharmacology for nurses, 13th edn. Edinburgh: Churchill Livingstone, 1999

SPC from the eMC, Piriton® tablets, Stafford-Miller Ltd, updated on the eMC June 2000

SPC from the eMC, Benadryl® Hayfever Relief, Warner Lambert Consumer Healthcare, updated on the eMC 28/08/01

SPC from the eMC, Clarityn®, Schering Plough Ltd, updated on the eMC 20/08/01

Stockley IH (ed) Drug interactions. London: Pharmaceutical Press, 1999

BP	CHLORPHENIRAMINE MALEATE
Proprietary	Piriton® (Stafford–Miller Ltd), Boots Allergy Relief Antihistamine tablets, Calimal® (Boots Company PLC), chlorpheniramine maleate (non-proprietary, see BNF)
Group	antihistamine – sedative
Uses/indications	urticaria, hayfever, allergic rhinitis, insect bites, drug allergies, **anaphylaxis**, food allergy, serum allergies
Type of drug	POM/GSL
Presentation	tablets, syrup, ampoules
Dosage	oral: 4 mg 4–6-hrly to a max. 24 mg daily
	s.c. or IM: 10–20 mg; repeat if required to a max. 40 mg in 24 hrs
	IV injection over 1 minute: 10–20 mg
Route of admin	oral, IM, slow IV injection (see chapter on emergency drugs)
Contraindications	epilepsy, hepatic disease, asthma as it has little effect on allergic bronchospasm, hypersensitivity
Side effects	drowsiness, lassitude, dizziness, dry mouth, blurred vision, headache, gastro-intestinal disturbances, IV may cause transient hypotension, CNS stimulation and may be an irritant, inability to concentrate, hepatitis – including jaundice, urinary retention, palpitations, arrhythmias, hypotension, chest tightness, blood disorders including haemolytic anaemia

table continues

	allergic reactions: exfoliative dermatitis, photosensitivity, twitching, urticaria, muscle weakness, inco-ordination, tinnitus, depression, irritability, nightmares
Interactions	*alcohol* – potentiates sedative action *antidepressants* – enhances sedative effect – anticholinergic effect intensified with MAOIs *antidiabetics* – depressed thrombocyte count *antiepileptics* – inhibits the metabolism of phenytoin *antihistamines* – concomitant therapy NOT recommended *anxiolytics and hypnotics* – enhance the sedative effect
Pharmacodynamic properties	potent antihistamine H_1 antagonist that antagonizes histamine-induced effects such as increased capillary permeability and the constriction of GI and respiratory smooth muscle. It is also a weak antimuscarinic and a moderate anti-serotonic, with local anaesthetic effect which can cause either CNS stimulation or depression
Fetal risk	no evidence of teratogenicity – manufacturers advise avoidance, as use in the third trimester may result in reactions in the neonate
Breastfeeding	considered moderately safe as secreted in significant amounts with no known effects, therefore avoidance is advised. It may also cause drowsiness in infants and inhibit lactation in mothers

Other antihistamines on the market which are used in the relief of allergies, including hayfever, are:

- Acrivastane – Benadryl® Hayfever Relief (Warner Lambert Consumer Healthcare)
- Terfenadine – non-proprietary, see BNF
- Loratadine – Clarityn® (Schering Plough Ltd), Boots Hayfever and Allergy Relief All Day® (Boots Company PLC)

ALL of the above are not recommended for use in pregnancy and the risk of embryotoxicity is high with loratadine and terfenadine

Chapter 13

Hypoglycaemics

These are agents that reduce the excessive level of glucose in the blood that is a feature of diabetes.

Insulin is a fuel-regulating hormone that controls the amount of glucose in the blood. Diabetics have a deficiency of insulin and therefore have a raised blood glucose level. There are three types of hypoglycaemic available: rapid acting, intermediate acting and long acting.

A medical diabetic consultant as well as a consultant obstetrician should care for women who have either insulin-dependent or gestational diabetes.

This chapter discusses the treatment used during pregnancy and does not address oral hypoglycaemics such as glibenclamide, as they are rarely used during pregnancy.

The student should be aware of:

- The physiology and pathophysiology of diabetes
- The treatment of diabetes
- The methods for diagnosing 'gestational diabetes' and methods of treating the condition
- The sequelae of a diabetic pregnancy
- Local protocols for the care and treatment of diabetic mothers during ante-, intra- and postpartum periods, and during operative procedures such as LSCS (lower-segment caesarean section)
- Care of the neonate after a diabetic pregnancy.

EXAMPLES OF INSULIN REGIMENS (SUBJECT TO ALTERATION ACCORDING TO INDIVIDUAL PATIENT REQUIREMENTS)

Short-acting insulin

Subcutaneous
- Usually administered 15–30 minutes before meals
- Effective after 30–60 minutes
- Peak effect after 2–4 hrs
- Duration 8 hrs.

NB: Human preparations have more rapid onset and shorter durations.

IV: half-life = 5 minutes and no longer effective after 30 minutes

Intermediate and long-acting insulin

Subcutaneous
- Onset 1–2 hrs
- Peak effect 4–12 hrs
- Duration 16–35 hrs.

Modified insulins such as biphasic isophane insulin, e.g. **Mixtard 30/70**®, or insulin zinc, e.g. **Human Monotard**®, mean that the insulin can be absorbed more slowly and act more smoothly. In pregnancy this is useful as dose adjustment may be required.

Insulin therapy is usually substituted for oral therapy in pregnancy and oral hypoglycaemics should not be used during breastfeeding.

References

Briggs GG, Freeman RK, Yaffe SJ. Drugs in pregnancy and lactation: a reference guide to fetal and neonatal risk, 3rd edn. Baltimore: Williams & Wilkins, 1990

British Medical Association and the Royal Pharmaceutical Society of Great Britain. British national formulary. Number 43, March 2002. Bath: Bath Press, 2002

Hale T. Medications and mothers' milk, 9th edn. USA: Pharmasoft Publications, 2000

Hopkins SJ. Drugs and pharmacology for nurses, 13th edn. Edinburgh: Churchill Livingstone, 1999

Landen MB, Gabbe SG. Diabetes in pregnancy. In: James DK, Steer PJ, Weiner CP, Gonik B (eds) High risk pregnancy: management options, 2nd edn. London: WB Saunders, 1999; 665–684

Little BB. Medication during pregnancy. In: James DK, Steer PJ, Weiner CP, Gonik B (eds) High risk pregnancy: management options, 2nd edn. London: WB Saunders, 1999; 617–638

SPC from the eMC, Human Actrapid®, Novo Nordisk Ltd, updated from the eMC, 22/08/01

SPC from the eMC, Novomix 30®, Novo Nordisk Ltd, updated from the eMC 08/05/02

SPC from the eMC, Human Mixtard®, Novo Nordisk Ltd, updated from the eMC 17/08/01

SPC from the eMC, Human Monotard®, Novo Nordisk Ltd, updated from the eMC 21/08/01

Stockley IH (ed) Drug interactions. London: Pharmaceutical Press, 1999

Acknowledgement

The author wishes to thank Jackie Maslin RGN, RM for her help in compiling this chapter.

BP	INSULIN ZINC SUSPENSION
Proprietary	Human Monotard® (Novo Nordisk Ltd)
Group	long-acting insulin
Uses/indications	insulin-dependent diabetes mellitus, insulin-dependent gestational diabetes
Type of drug	POM
Presentation	ampoules, pre-filled pen syringes
Dosage	according to agreed regimen and patient requirements, usually used once daily, e.g. in the evening and/or in the morning, it can be used alone or with a short-acting insulin at meals, effective within 22 hrs, peak effect 7–15 hrs, duration 24 hrs
Route of admin	subcutaneous
Contraindications	as for soluble insulin
Side effects	as for soluble insulin
Interactions	as for soluble insulin
Pharmacodynamic properties	as for soluble insulin
Fetal risk	as for soluble insulin
Breastfeeding	as for soluble insulin

BP	BIPHASIC ISOPHANE INSULIN – SUSPENSION OF INSULIN IN PROTAMINE
Proprietary	Human Mixtard® (various concentrations) (Novo Nordisk Ltd), Humulin M3® (Lilly), Humulin M5® (Lilly)
Group	intermediate-acting insulins
Uses/indications	insulin-dependent diabetes mellitus, insulin-dependent gestational diabetes, has value in initiation of b.d. insulin regimens
Type of drug	POM
Presentation	ampoules, pre-prepared cartridges/pens
Dosage	usually b.d. when a rapid initial effect with prolonged effect is required, according to agreed regimen and according to patient requirements, followed by meal/snack of carbohydrates in 30 minutes, effective within 30 minutes, peak effect 2–8 hrs, duration 24 hrs
Route of admin	subcutaneous
Contraindications	as for soluble insulin, hypersensitivity to protamine
Side effects	hypoglycaemia, protamine can cause an allergic reaction, fat hypertrophy at injection sites
Interactions	as for soluble insulin
Pharmacodynamic properties	as for soluble insulin
Fetal risk	as for soluble insulin
Breastfeeding	as for soluble insulin

BP	SOLUBLE INSULINS
Proprietary	Human Actrapid® (Novo Nordisk Ltd), Novo Nordisk 30® (Novo Nordisk Ltd), Humulin® (Lilly)
Group	short-acting insulin
Uses/indications	insulin-dependent diabetes mellitus, diabetic ketoacidosis, insulin-dependent gestational diabetes
Type of drug	POM
Presentation	ampoules, preprepared cartridges
Dosage	according to agreed regimen and according to patient requirements, 30 minutes prior to or soon after meal, effective within 10–20 minutes of dose, max. effect 1–4 hrs, duration 24 hrs
Route of admin	subcutaneous, IM, IV injection/infusion
Contraindications	reduce dosage in renal impairment
Side effects	hypoglycaemia, local reactions, fat hypertrophy at injection sites
Interactions	*alcohol* – enhances the hypoglycaemic effect *analgesics* – salicylates increase insulin requirements *antidepressants* – MAOIs increase insulin requirements *β-blockers* – enhances hypoglycaemic effect and masks the warning signs, i.e. tremor *corticosteroids* – antagonize the hypoglycaemic effect

table continues

	contraceptives – antagonize the hypoglycaemic effect *nifedipine* – may cause impaired glucose tolerance
Pharmacodynamic properties	the blood glucose-lowering effect of insulin is due to the binding of insulin to receptors on fat and muscle cells and a simultaneous inhibition of glucose output from the liver
Fetal risk	insulin is an antagonist to surfactant production, some evidence of fetal growth deficiency, frequent antenatal surveillance is recommended. Insulin does not cross the placental barrier and requirements fall in the first trimester and rise subsequently in the second and third trimesters. After delivery requirements return rapidly to prepregnancy values if the diabetes is poorly controlled. US studies have reported a 2–4-fold greater probability of congenital defects induced prior to 7 weeks' gestation, and these are usually responsible for the higher rate of first-trimester abortions among this patient group
Breastfeeding	insulin is a natural constituent of blood and is not secreted in breast milk; however, insulin dosage may need to be reduced

Chapter 14

Intravenous Fluids

These are solutions of electrolytes which may be used as carriers or as described to maintain the electrolyte balance of the body when intra- or extracellular water changes occur, e.g. in haemorrhage, dehydration or ketoacidosis.

Plasma expanders are used when there is sudden acute blood or plasma loss leading to a fall in blood pressure and the remaining blood cells collapse to try to redress the balance.

Drugs should NOT be added to infusions of sodium bicarbonate, amino acids, mannitol, blood products or specially prepared fat emulsions such as are used in neonatal intensive care units for feeding neonates (total parenteral nutrition) via the intravenous route.

Instructions as to storage and degradation of solutions should be noted, and any deviation either from instructions or within the solution should indicate that stopping the infusion is necessary.

Additive labels should be used to indicate what has been added to the solution, time, strength and, if relevant, expiry time/date, as well as patient identity and the signature of the practitioners checking the infusion. The practitioner must also be aware of the suitability of the additive to the electrolyte solution and where to refer any enquiries.

INTRAVENOUS FLUIDS IN COMMON USE

Sodium chloride 0.9% – isotonic solution – used in fluid replacement and electrolyte balance as an IV infusion, as a carrier for injections in which the prescribed drug requires reconstitution, or as a 'flush' for IV cannulae.

Glucose 5% – used as an intravenous infusion (IVI) for fluid replacement and balance, where there is dehydration without severe electrolyte loss, and also when there is an insulin infusion for the prevention of diabetic ketoacidosis, i.e. during diabetic labours.

Dextrose saline – sodium chloride 0.18 % + glucose 4% – contra-indicated in hyperemesis due to increased risk of Wernicke's encephalopathy – if necessary to balance electrolytes then give thiamine first and refer to BNF for dosage.

Hartmann's Solution (compound sodium lactate solution) – isotonic solution – used as IVI to replace fluid and restore electrolyte balance, often used in obstetrics as a carrier for syntocinon infusions or for 'preloading' prior to and during epidural analgesia.

Water for injection – used to reconstitute drugs prescribed as IVI injection.

Potassium chloride + glucose – used in severe electrolyte depletion – should be used with caution as rapid infusion is toxic to the heart; exact regimen specified by the prescriber.

Potassium chloride + sodium chloride – as above.

Potassium chloride + glucose + sodium chloride – as above, specified by the prescriber.

PLASMA EXPANDERS

Haemaccel® (Beacon), Gelofusine® (Braun) – used when there is low blood volume, and after an initial 500–1000 mL further doses are given depending on the patient's condition.

References

British Medical Association and the Royal Pharmaceutical Society of Great Britain. British national formulary. Number 43, March 2002. Bath: Bath Press, 2002

Hopkins SJ. Drugs and pharmacology for nurses, 13th edn. Edinburgh: Churchill Livingstone, 1999

SPC from the eMC, Haemaccel®, Beacon Pharmaceuticals, updated on the eMC 16/07/01

Chapter 15

Immunoglobulins

These are antibodies, present in the blood, which by specific and direct action defend the body against invading bacteria or organisms. The anti-D immunoglobulin is used in the treatment of rhesus iso-immunization in women whose blood is rhesus negative. This immunoglobulin, given via injection, coats the fetal cells that may have leaked into the maternal circulation following a sensitizing episode, thus preventing the woman becoming rhesus iso-immunized.

Some antibodies that are present in maternal blood require consultation with Regional Blood Transfusion Centres as to their relevance to the mother and the fetus/neonate.

Other uses of immunoglobulins include those used as vaccines, i.e. hepatitis, rabies and tetanus.

The student should be aware of:

- Blood grouping and rhesus evaluation
- The aetiology of Rhesus iso-immunization
- Prevention of iso-immunization
- What action should be taken when there is a possibility that iso-immunization could occur, e.g. in antepartum haemorrhage
- Counselling to prevent iso-immunization
- The sequlae to mother and fetus/neonate of Rhesus iso-immunization
- The RCOG and NICE guidelines for administration of anti-D in pregnancy

- An awareness of other antibodies present in blood, e.g. Lewis, Kell, Duffy anti-E and anti-Fy etc.
- The sequelae of infection by varicella zoster in pregnant mothers and neonates
- The administration of immunoglobulin to ameliorate the effects of such infection
- The RCOG guidelines for treatment of varicella zoster contacts.

When evaluating titres the date of the last dose of anti-D should be included as the antibodies persist in circulation and may give a falsely high reading.

Rubella vaccine can also be administered in the postpartum period with anti-D provided that separate syringes are used and they are administered in contralateral (opposite side) limbs. If blood transfusion was necessary then rubella vaccination should delayed for 3 months.

MMR vaccine should NOT be given within 3 months of anti-D immunoglobulin.

References

British Medical Association and the Royal Pharmaceutical Society of Great Britain. British national formulary. Number 43, March 2002. Bath: Bath Press, 2002

Hale T. Medications and mothers' milk, 9th edn. USA: Pharmasoft Publications, 2000

Hopkins SJ. Drugs and pharmacology for nurses, 13th edn. Edinburgh: Churchill Livingstone, 1999

National Institute for Clinical Excellence. Guidance on the use of routine antenatal anti-D prophylaxis for RhD-negative women. Technology Appraisal Guidance No.41, May 2002

Royal College of Obstetricians and Gynaecologists. Use of anti-D immunoglobulin for rhesus prophylaxis. Clinical Greentop Guidelines No.22, October 1999

Royal College of Obstetricians and Gynaecologists. Chickenpox in pregnancy. Clinical Greentop Guidelines No.13, July 2001

SPC from the eMC, Anti-D (RHO) immunoglobulin injection BP, Baxter Healthcare Ltd, updated on the eMC 07/04/03

SPC from the eMC, Rophylac®, 300 (1500 i.u.), updated on the eMC 03/10/03

SPC from the eMC, Varilrix®, SmithKline Beecham UK, updated on the eMC 02/08/02

BP	ANTI-D (RH) IMMUNOGLOBULIN
Proprietary	Anti-D Rh Immunoglobulin (BPL), also Anti-D (RHO) Immunoglobulin Injection BP® (Baxter Healthcare Ltd)
Group	immunoglobulins – specific
Uses/indications	to prevent rhesus iso-immunization
Type of drug	POM
Presentation	pre-prepared vials, preloaded syringes
Dosage	after any potentially sensitizing episode, e.g. vaginal bleeding of uterine origin, abortion or amniocentesis up to 20 weeks' gestation: 250 units per episode (within 72 hrs) following sensitizing episode after 20 weeks, e.g. birth of Rhesus–positive infant, antepartum haemorrhage: 500 units (within 72 hrs) dosage may vary according to the titre of fetal cells detected.
	NICE guidelines (2002) recommend that all women who are Rhesus D-negative be given anti-D at 28 and 34 weeks gestation
Route of admin	deep IM
Contraindications	caution in those who have had an adverse reaction to blood transfusion or to administration of blood derivatives
Side effects	soreness at injection site

table continues

Interactions	*live vaccines* – if anti-D is given within 2–4 weeks of live vaccine then its action may be impaired
Pharmacodynamic properties	during a sensitizing episode when fetal cells enter the maternal circulation, if they are Rhesus D positive then the body treats them as foreign and makes antibodies against them. This is iso-immunization. When the mother comes into contact with Rhesus-D positive cells again, either later in the same pregnancy or in subsequent pregnancies, then her immune system produces immunoglobulins that cross the placenta and destroy fetal blood cells, causing haemolytic disease in the fetus. Anti-D coats fetal cells and disguises them from the maternal immune system so that either the mother remains non-immunized or her system is 'blind' to the fetal cells until they degrade naturally
Fetal risk	N/A
Breastfeeding	no data available

BP	VARICELLA ZOSTER IMMUNOGLOBULIN
Proprietary	VZIG immunoglobulin (BPL), Varilrix® (SmithKline Beecham UK)
Group	immunoglobulins – specific
Uses/indications	against varicella in healthy adults who are seronegative to the varicella zoster virus, including neonates of women who develop chickenpox within 7 days before and after delivery
Type of drug	POM
Presentation	powder and solvent to prepare solution for injection, vials of solution for injection
Dosage	Varilrix: 2 ampoules/solution for injection, each containing 0.5 mL of reconstituted virus – interval between doses should be 8 weeks, but minimum 6 weeks BPL dosage: deep IM – not later than 10 days after exposure – 1g. If there is further exposure then repeat dose of 1g 3 weeks after the first
Route of admin	s.c.
Contraindications	hypersensitivity to neomycin, those in an immuno-compromised state, pregnancy and breastfeeding
Side effects	acquiring chicken pox, headache, dizziness, nausea, muscle aches
Interactions	

table continues

Pharmacodynamic properties	infection of the subject with varicella zoster induces the humoral and cell-mediated immune response and thus immunity
Fetal risk	Exposure in utero may cause the fetus to contract chickenpox, and it can then be born with either a mild dose form of chickenpox or scars from lesions acquired during infection. Causes problems with the respiratory tract
Breastfeeding	considered safe

Chapter 16

Oxytocics

Oxytocics are drugs used to stimulate uterine contractions, to augment labour, to expedite delivery of the fetus, and in the third stage the delivery of the placenta and to halt postpartum haemorrhage.

The student should be aware of:

- The physiology of labour
- Reasons for prolonged, incoordinate labour/contractions
- The physical, psychological and chemical factors that could diminish contractions
- Reasons to expedite delivery
- Research pertaining to managed and physiological third stage of labour
- Appropriate emergency action to be taken in the event of syntocinon overdose
- The local emergency protocol for postpartum haemorrhage
- The sequelae of oxytocin administration in mother and neonate
- Local protocols for the induction and augmentation of labour, including contra-indications to therapy, e.g. cord prolapse, cephalo-pelvic disproportion, malpresentation, placenta praevia, antepartum haemorrhage, and cautions in predisposition to uterine rupture, multiple pregnancy, grande multiparity, polyhydramnios, previous caesarean section
- The action of oxytocin, ergometrine and syntometrine.

References

Briggs GG, Freeman RK, Yaffe SJ. Drugs in pregnancy and lactation: a reference guide to fetal and neonatal risk, 3rd edn. Baltimore: Williams & Wilkins, 1990

British Medical Association and the Royal Pharmaceutical Society of Great Britain. British national formulary. Number 43, March 2002. Bath: Bath Press, 2002

Hale T. Medications and mothers' milk, 9th edn. USA: Pharmasoft Publications, 2000

Hopkins SJ. Drugs and pharmacology for nurses, 13th edn. Edinburgh: Churchill Livingstone, 1999

Little BB. Medication during pregnancy. In: James DK, Steer PJ, Weiner CP, Gonik B (eds) High risk pregnancy: management options, 2nd edn. London: WB Saunders, 1999; 617–638

National Institute for Clinical Excellence. Induction of labour. Inherited Clinical Guideline D, June 2001

Shiers CV. Prolonged pregnancy and disorders of uterine action. In: Bennett VR, Brown LK (eds) Myles textbook for midwives, 13th edn. Edinburgh: Churchill Livingstone, 1999; 489–506

SPC from the eMC, Syntocinon®, Alliance Pharmaceuticals, updated on the eMC 07/08/01

SPC from the eMC, Syntometrine®, Alliance Pharmaceuticals, updated on the eMC 16/07/01

SPC from the eMC, Ergometrine® tablets, Celltech Manufacturing Services Ltd, updated on the eMC 07/02/02

Stockley IH (ed) Drug interactions. London: Pharmaceutical Press, 1999

BP	ERGOMETRINE MALEATE
Proprietary	Ergometrine® tablets (Celltech), ergometrine (non-proprietary, see BNF)
Group	oxytocic-like substance
Uses/indications	postpartum haemorrhage (rarely used)
Type of drug.	POM
Presentation	ampoules, tablets
Dosage	IM: 200–500 µg (ampoules can be given orally when no access to syringe and needle, but this is very rare and not recommended – effective in 10 minutes according to BNF) oral: 0.5–1 mg
Route of admin	IM, oral
Contraindications	pregnancy, first and second stages of labour, as for syntometrine, hypertension, hypersensitivity to ergometrine, i.e. previous ergotism
Side effects	as for syntometrine
Interactions	
Pharmacodynamic properties	causes the uterine smooth muscle to contract, producing a sustained uterine contraction, in contrast to the rhythmic physiological contractions produced by oxytocin. It causes vasoconstriction in peripheral blood vessels but can affect the major blood vessels

table continues

Fetal risk	ABORTIFACIENT
Breastfeeding	limited data available on breastfeeding women but considered moderately safe and is secreted in breast milk

BP	ERGOMETRINE MALEATE WITH OXYTOCIN
Proprietary	Syntometrine® (Alliance)
Group	oxytocic
Uses/indications	to expedite placental delivery, to control haemorrhage
Type of drug	POM
Presentation	ampoules
Dosage	one ampoule: ergometrine 500 µg + 5 units oxytocin in 1 mL
Route of admin	IM
Contraindications	pre-eclampsia, renal impairment, first and second stages of labour, hepatic, cardiac or pulmonary disease, previous adverse reaction
Side effects	nausea, vomiting, headache, dizziness, tinnitus, chest pain, palpitations, vasoconstriction, myocardial infarction, pulmonary oedema, stroke
Interactions	
Pharmacodynamic properties	combines the sustained oxytocic action of ergometrine with the rapid action of oxytocin to act on the smooth muscle of the uterus to expedite placental separation and to control bleeding from the site of placentation after delivery
Fetal risk	causes sustained uterine contraction and restriction of placental blood flow, leading to lack of oxygen to the fetus. If given to

table continues

	the neonate by accident causes serious and possibly fatal multi-organ shutdown
Breastfeeding	as for ergometrine

BP	OXYTOCIN
Proprietary	Syntocinon® (Alliance)
Group	oxytocic
Uses/indications	augmentation/induction of labour, control of postpartum haemorrhage
Type of drug.	POM
Presentation	ampoules (5 units, 10 units)
Dosage	according to protocol
Route of admin	IM, IVI or slow IV injection
Contraindications	not within 6 hrs of prostaglandin administration, intact membranes, hypertonic uterine contractions, mechanical obstruction to delivery, fetal distress, where vaginal delivery is inadvisable, oxytocin-resistant uterine inertia, placenta praevia, vasa praevia, placental abruption, cord presentation or prolapse, severe pre-eclampsia, cardiovascular disease, caution in grande multiparity or where there is predisposition to uterine rupture, polyhydramnios, in cases of IUD or meconium-stained liquor – avoid tumultuous labour as it may cause amniotic fluid embolism
Side effects	uterine spasm, uterine hyperstimulation, antidiuretic causing water intoxication, hypernatraemia, nausea, vomiting, rashes, **anaphylaxis**, placental abruption, amniotic fluid embolism – exclude diagnosis prior to beginning therapy

table continues

Interactions	*anaesthetics* – can potentiate the hypotensive effect and may cause arrhythmias; the oxytocic effect may be reduced
	prostaglandins – uterotonic effect potentiated
Pharmacodynamic properties	synthetic form of the hormone oxytocin. It exerts a stimulatory effect on uterine smooth muscle, especially at the end of pregnancy, during labour and post delivery, and in the puerperium when receptors in the myometrium are increased. In low doses it causes rhythmic contractions but in high doses it causes hypertonic, sustained contractions
Fetal risk	fetal distress, asphyxia, IUD (intrauterine death), infusions in labour may be associated with neonatal jaundice
Breastfeeding	considered safe

Chapter 17

Prostaglandins

Prostaglandins are hormones secreted by various body tissues, e.g. uterine and cardiac muscle, semen and the lungs.

In obstetrics prostaglandins are used to ripen the uterine cervix and cause contractions during the induction of labour.

Students should be aware of:

- The indications for induction of labour
- Local protocols for induction of labour – specifically the dosage used
- The action of prostaglandins with respect to termination of pregnancy and the side effects
- The use of the Bishop's Score in the induction of labour.

References

British Medical Association and the Royal Pharmaceutical Society of Great Britain. British national formulary. Number 43, March 2002. Bath: Bath Press, 2002

Hale T. Medications and mothers'milk, 9th edn. USA: Pharmasoft Publications, 2000

Hopkins SJ. Drugs and pharmacology for nurses, 13th edn. Edinburgh: Churchill Livingstone, 1999

Little BB. Medication during pregnancy. In: James DK, Steer PJ, Weiner CP, Gonik B (eds) High risk pregnancy: management options, 2nd edn. London: WB Saunders, 1999; 617–638

Shiers CV. Prolonged pregnancy and disorders of uterine action. In: Bennett VR, Brown LK (eds) Myles textbook for midwives, 13th edn. Edinburgh: Churchill Livingstone, 1999; 489–506

SPC from the eMC, Prostin E2® vaginal gel 1 mg/2 mg, Pharmacia, updated on the eMC 03/10/01

SPC from the eMC, Prostin E2® vaginal tablets, Pharmacia, updated on the eMC 24/08/01

SPC from the eMC, Gemeprost®, Beacon Pharmaceuticals, updated on the eMC 14/01/02

Stockley IH (ed) Drug interactions. London: Pharmaceutical Press, 1999

BP	GEMEPROST
Proprietary	Gemeprost® (non-proprietary see BNF)
Group	prostaglandin
Uses/indications	used in cervical ripening during therapeutic termination
Type of drug	POM
Presentation	pessaries
Dosage	dependent on stage of pregnancy and indication
Route of admin	per vaginam
Contraindications	chronic obstructive airways disease, cardiovascular insufficiency, raised intraocular pressure, cervicitis, vaginitis; caution should be used with previous uterine surgery
Side effects	vaginal bleeding, uterine pain, nausea, vomiting, diarrhoea, headache, flushing, chills, dizziness, muscle weakness, backache, dyspnoea, chest pain, mild pyrexia, uterine rupture especially with previous LSCS, grande multiparity
Interactions	*oxytocics* – enhances uterotonic effect
Pharmacodynamic properties	a prostaglandin of the E_1 series that causes uterine contractions, softening, and a decrease in the resistance of cervical tissue. It also depresses placental and uterine blood flow, secondary to uterine contractions
Fetal risk	**ABORTIFACIENT**
Breastfeeding	not applicable

BP	DINOPROSTONE
Proprietary	Prostin E2® (Pharmacia)
Group	prostaglandins
Uses/indications	induction of labour – ripening of the cervix for labour
Type of drug	POM
Presentation	vaginal gel or pessaries (rarely used – tablets, IV solution, extra-amniotic solution)
Dosage	CAUTION – Prostin E2 gel is not a bioequivalent to Prostin E2 tablets dependent on parity, local protocols and Bishop's Score repeated 6-hrly maximum dosage refers to amount given at each attempt to induce labour, not to each dose given gel max. dose = 3 mg (4 mg in unfavourable primiparae) tablet max. dose = 6 mg in primiparae, less in multiparae
Route of admin	per vaginam (not intracervical)
Contraindications	previous sensitivity, cephalo-pelvic disproportion, ruptured membranes, previous caesarean section or uterine surgery, untreated pelvic infection, grande multiparity, fetal distress, avoid in cervicitis or vaginitis, active cardiac, pulmonary, renal or hepatic disease, placenta praevia, unexplained vaginal bleeding

table continues

	CAUTION: asthma, cardiac, hepatic or renal impairment, hypertension, history of epilepsy, uterine scarring
Side effects	nausea, vomiting, diarrhoea, severe uterine contractions, overdosage leading to uterine rupture, uterine hypertonus, pulmonary or amniotic fluid embolism, abruptio placentae, maternal hypotension, bronchospasm, fever, backache, rapid cervical dilation, hypercontractility with or without fetal distress, low Apgar scores, cardiac arrest, stillbirth, neonatal death
	vaginal symptoms: warmth, irritation, pain after dose, flushing, sweating, headache, dizziness, temporary pyrexia
Interactions	*oxytocics* – uterotonic effect enhanced
Pharmacodynamic properties	a prostaglandin of the E_2 series which induces myometrial contractions and promotes cervical ripening
Fetal risk	**ABORTIFACIENT**. Exposure to fetal skin in utero causes fetal heart rate abnormalities and may predispose to neonatal jaundice
Breastfeeding	considered moderately safe, but with extremely limited data on the consequences of administration in breastfeeding women

Chapter 18

Myometrial Relaxants

These drugs are sympathomimetics and relax uterine muscle, hopefully preventing premature labour. Mostly they are used to delay delivery until corticosteroid therapy is complete. Some are used as antagonists to oxytocin hyperstimulation of the uterus during the induction or augmentation of labour. Their use is indicated between 24 and 34 weeks gestation in uncomplicated cases.

The student should be aware of:

- What constitutes premature labour
- Local protocols for the management of premature labour
- The sequelae of the action of these drugs on the mother and fetus.

References

Briggs GG, Freeman RK, Yaffe SJ. Drugs in pregnancy and lactation: a reference guide to fetal and neonatal risk, 3rd edn. Baltimore: Williams & Wilkins, 1990

British Medical Association and the Royal Pharmaceutical Society of Great Britain. British national formulary. Number 43, March 2002. Bath: Bath Press, 2002

Hale T. Medications and mothers' milk, 9th edn. USA: Pharmasoft Publications, 2000

Hopkins SJ. Drugs and pharmacology for nurses, 13th edn. Edinburgh: Churchill Livingstone, 1999

Little BB. Medication during pregnancy. In: James DK, Steer PJ, Weiner CP, Gonik B (eds) High risk pregnancy: management options, 2nd edn. London: WB Saunders, 1999; 617–638

Lloyd C, Lewis VM. Common medical disorders associated with pregnancy. In: Bennett VR, Brown LK (eds) Myles textbook for midwives, 13th edn. Edinburgh: Churchill Livingstone, 1999; 279–314

Royal College of Obstetricians and Gynaecologists. Beta-agonists for the care of women in preterm labour. Clinical Greentop Guidelines No.1A. June 1997, reviewed February 2000

Royal College of Obstetricians and Gynaecologists. Tocolytic drugs for women in preterm labour. Clinical Greentop Guidelines No 1B. October 2002

SPC from the eMC, Yutopar®, Solvay Healthcare Ltd, updated on the eMC 05/03/02

SPC from the eMC, Ventolin™, Allen & Hanburys, updated on the eMC 25/03/02

SPC from the eMC, Bricanyl®, AstraZeneca, updated on the eMC 07/06/02

SPC from the eMC, Bricanyl® tablets and syrup, AstraZeneca, updated on the eMC 09/07/02

SPC from the eMC, Adalat®, Bayer PLC, updated on the eMC 16/08/01

Stockley IH (ed) Drug interactions. London: Pharmaceutical Press, 1999)

http://www.wholehealthmd.com/refshelf/drugs – pharmacodynamic properties of nifedipine

BP	TERBUTALINE
Proprietary	Bricanyl® injection (AstraZeneca)
Group	myometrial relaxant/bronchodilator
Uses/indications	inhibition of uncomplicated labour 24–33 weeks' gestation – as for ritodrine
Type of drug	POM
Presentation	ampoules, tablets
Dosage	as per local protocols or the SPC – use of syringe pump or controlled infusion device essential
Route of admin	IVI, subcutaneous, IM, oral
Contraindications	as for ritodrine
Side effects	as for salbutamol and ritodrine
Interactions	as for ritodrine
Pharmacodynamic properties	selective β_2-adrenergic stimulant that inhibits uterine contractility
Fetal risk	as for ritodrine
Breastfeeding	secreted in breast milk but amounts are too small to be harmful

BP	SALBUTAMOL
Proprietary	Ventolin™ for IV infusion (Allen and Hanburys), non-proprietary, see BNF for details
Group	myometrial relaxant/bronchodilator
Uses/indications	inhibition of uncomplicated premature labour 24–33 weeks' gestation, also used to antagonize hypertonic contractions
Type of drug	POM
Presentation	ampoules, syrup, tablets, inhalers
Dosage	syringe pump or controlled infusion device essential
	IV dosage: as per local protocols, for example 10–45 µg/min. Stat 10 µg increased at 10-minute intervals until response of diminution of strength/frequency/duration of contractions, then slowly increase until contractions cease. Maintain for 1 hr then decrease by 50% decrements 6-hrly. If contractions have ceased use Ventolin tablets 4 mg t.d.s./q.d.s.
Route of admin	oral, IM, IV/infusion (in 5% dextrose – can use NaCl with diabetic patients)
Contraindications	as for ritodrine – caution with diabetics
Side effects	fine tremor, tension, headache, peripheral vasodilation, tachycardia if over 140 bpm – cease infusion, hypersensitivity, pulmonary oedema – observe the volume of fluid infused

table continues

Interactions	as for ritodrine
Pharmacodynamic properties	a selective β-antagonist which acts upon receptors in the uterus and bronchi, causing them to relax and lessening contractility
Fetal risk	unknown safety, in animals teratogenicity during early gestation, otherwise as for ritodrine
Breastfeeding	evidence for the safety of salbutamol during lactation – not conclusive

BP	RITODRINE HYDROCHLORIDE
Proprietary	Yutopar® (Solvay Healthcare Ltd)
Group	myometrial relaxant
Uses/indications	inhibition of uncomplicated premature labour between 24 and 33 weeks' gestation, or to delay delivery by up to 48 hrs to administer glucocorticosteroids and implement other measures for neonatal wellbeing. Less effective if cervix 4 cm dilated or rupture of membranes is confirmed
Type of drug	POM
Presentation	ampoules, tablets (yellow) used to maintain uterine quiescence only
Dosage	as per local protocols, syringe pump or controlled infusion device is essential, for example IVI: initial 50 µg/min, increased according to response by 50 µg/min every 10 minutes until the contractions stop or the maternal pulse reaches 140 bpm, or max. dose of 350 µg/min usually effective between 150 and 350 µg/min – always use the lowest effective dose and continue at that dose for 12–48 hrs after the contractions cease
	in uterine hypertonicity: 50 µg/min IV until the uterus relaxes
	oral: 10 mg tablet 30 minutes prior to ceasing infusion, then 10–20 mg every 2–6 hrs depending on uterine activity and the side effects. The dose should not

table continues

	exceed 120 mg/day and should continue as long as it is desirable to maintain the pregnancy
Route of admin	oral, IM, IV (in 5% dextrose)
Contraindications	if labour progresses after the maximum 350 µg dose, cord compression, chorioamnitis, cardiac disease, pre-eclampsia, eclampsia, intrauterine infection, intrauterine death, obstetric haemorrhage, placenta praevia, first and second trimesters of pregnancy
Side effects	nausea, vomiting, sweating, tremor, tachycardia if over 140 bpm – cease infusion, palpitations, hypotension, increased tendency to uterine bleeding, pulmonary oedema, chest pain and tightness, *use caution with hydration and if pulmonary oedema develops cease infusion* predisposing factors are fluid overload, multiple pregnancy, cardiac disease and maternal infection
Interactions	*anaesthetics* – potential hypotensive effect *β–blockers* – inhibit the action of ritodrine *corticosteroids* – with a high dose of ritodrine and high dose of corticosteroids there is an increased risk of hypokalaemia *loop diuretics and thiazides* – risk of hypokalaemia *sympathomimetics* – concurrent use potentiates the effects of ritodrine *theophylline* – risk of hypokalaemia

table continues

	CAUTION – when used IV in diabetic clients glucose levels should be monitored and insulin regimens need adjusting accordingly
Pharmacodynamic properties	a β-mimetic which stimulates β_2 receptors, thereby reducing uterine contractility. It also acts to cause cardiac effects and peripheral vasodilation at therapeutic doses
Fetal risk	increased risk of obstetric haemorrhage, intrauterine death, transient neonatal tachycardia failed to show teratogenicity but recommended to avoid during the first 16 weeks of gestation
Breastfeeding	considered moderately safe but limited data available

BP	NIFEDIPINE
Proprietary	Adalat® (Bayer), Nifedipine (non-proprietary see BNF)
Group	calcium channel blocker, hypotensive, vasodilator
Uses/indications	myometrial relaxant
Type of drug	POM
Presentation	capsules, tablets (slow release)
Dosage	10 mg stat. sublingually then 10 mg at 15-minute intervals for 1 hr or until contractions have ceased, then 60–120 mg/day via slow-release tablets (or as per local protocol) (maintenance dose 20–40 mg q.d.s.) max. dosage 160 mg in 24 hrs
Route of admin	oral
Contraindications	continuous use in pregnancy, breastfeeding, hypersensitivity, pre-eclampsia, pre-existing hypotension with systolic below 90 mmHg, previous adverse reaction to calcium channel blockers, cardiac disease – congestive cardiac failure, hepatic dysfunction, aortic stenosis
Side effects	headache, palpitations, flushing, dizziness, oedema, hypotension, nausea and vomiting CAUTION: stop treatment if ischaemic pain occurs within 30–60 minutes of administration.

table continues

	Treatment with short-acting nifedipine, i.e. during a crisis, can induce an exaggerated fall in blood pressure and reflex tachycardia, which may cause complications such as cerebrovascular accident/ischaemia or myocardial ischaemia
	Rarely: abnormal liver function tests, congestive cardiac failure, transient hypoglycaemia, tachycardia, chest pain, ischaemia (retinal/cerebral), tinnitus, pruritus
	EXTREME CAUTION when using magnesium sulphate
Interactions	do not take with grapefruit juice *antihypertensives* – causes severe hypotension and possible heart failure *cimetidine* – potentiates the hypotensive effect as metabolism of nifedipine is inhibited *phenytoin* – concomitant administration can reduce the effect of nifedipine – monitor plasma levels of anticonvulsants *erythromycin* – may potentiate nifedipine effects *insulin* – possible impaired glucose tolerance
Pharmacodynamic properties	a selective calcium channel blocker with mostly vascular effects. It is a specific and potent calcium antagonist which relaxes arterial smooth muscle, causing arteries to widen and reducing the resistance in coronary and peripheral circulation. This reduces blood pressure and decreases the heart's overall workload

table continues

Fetal risk	toxicity in animals, hypotensive effect can reduce placental flow and cause decrease in fetal oxygenation, i.e. *there is the potential for fetal hypoxia in association with maternal hypotension* contraindicated in suspected uterine infection, labour in the presence of placenta praevia, severe intrauterine growth retardation, lethal anomalies or fetal death in utero
Breastfeeding	considered safe 3–4 hrs after dose, but manufacturer advises avoidance

Chapter **19**

Rectal Preparations

LAXATIVES

These are medicines that loosen the bowel content and encourage evacuation. They are also known as aperients.

HAEMORRHOID PREPARATIONS

These come in the form of suppositories or topical creams and contain local anaesthetics or corticosteroids.

The student should be aware of:

- The effect of progesterone on the alimentary tract musculature
- Factors predisposing to haemorrhoids
- The use of dietary measures to alleviate constipation.

Haemorrhoid preparations

Haemorrhoid preparations are combinations of ingredients such as soothing compounds, e.g. local anaesthetic, and corticosteroids, e.g. hydrocortisone to alleviate the local inflammatory response; they may also contain mild astringents, vasoconstrictors and heparinoids to help relieve the haemorrhoid.

Anusol® – cream, ointment, suppositories – applied twice daily after a bowel movement, or one suppository twice daily – use neither for longer than 7 days

Scheriproct® – ointment or suppositories – apply twice daily for 5–7 days (3–4 times daily on first day if necessary), then once daily for a few days until symptoms have cleared, or one suppository daily after bowel movement for 5–7 days

Proctosedyl® – ointment or suppositories – apply twice daily after bowel movement, or insert one suppository twice daily after bowel movement – do not use either for longer than 7 days.

References

Briggs GG, Freeman RK, Yaffe SJ. Drugs in pregnancy and lactation: a reference guide to fetal and neonatal risk, 3rd edn. Baltimore: Williams & Wilkins, 1990

British Medical Association and the Royal Pharmaceutical Society of Great Britain. British national formulary. Number 43, March 2002. Bath: Bath Press, 2002

Hale T. Medications and mothers' milk, 9th edn. USA: Pharmasoft Publications, 2000

Hopkins SJ. Drugs and pharmacology for nurses, 13th edn. Edinburgh: Churchill Livingstone, 1999

SPC from the eMC, DulcoLax® suppositories 10 mg and DulcoLax® tablets 5 mg, Boehringer Ingelheim Ltd, Self Medication Division. Updated on the eMC 16/08/01

SPC from the eMC, Norgalax Micro-Enema®, Norgine Ltd, updated on the eMC 14/08/01

SPC from the eMC, glycerin suppositories, BP Boots Company PLC, updated on the eMC 04/03/02

SPC from the eMC, Senokot®, Britannia Pharmaceuticals Ltd, updated on the eMC 28/08/01

SPC from the eMC, Duphalac®, Solvay Healthcare Ltd updated from the eMC 05/07/01

SPC from the eMC, Lactulose Solution BP, Novartis Consumer Health, updated on the eMC 13/08/01

SPC from the eMC, Anusol® suppositories, ointment and cream, Warner Lambert Consumer Healthcare, updated on the eMC 24/08/01

SPC from the eMC Scheriproct® ointment and suppositories, Solvay Healthcare Ltd, updated on, the eMC 13/07/01

SPC from the eMC, Proctosedyl® ointment and suppositories, Aventis Pharma Ltd, updated on the eMC 06/01/02

BP	BISACODYL
Proprietary	Dulcolax® (Boehringer Ingelheim Ltd)
Group	stimulant laxative
Uses/indications	constipation
Type of drug	POM.
Presentation	tablets (white), suppositories
Dosage	5–10 mg nocte, action over 10–12 hrs
Route of admin	oral, p.r.
Contraindications	avoid in children
Side effects	abdominal cramps, not for prolonged use as it can cause atonic non-functioning colon and hypokalaemia
Interactions	no data available
Fetal risk	no data available
Breastfeeding	considered safe

BP	DOCUSATE SODIUM
Proprietary	Norgalax Micro-Enema® (Norgine Ltd)
Group	stimulant laxative
Uses/indications	constipation
Type of drug	POM
Presentation	enema
Dosage	120 mg in 10 g – single-dose disposable pack
Route of admin	p.r.
Contraindications	haemorrhoids, anal fissure
Side effects	local irritant
Interactions	N/A
Fetal risk	N/A
Breastfeeding	considered safe as transfer to breast milk minimal

BP	SENNA
Proprietary	Senokot® (Britannia Pharmaceuticals Ltd)
Group	stimulant laxatives
Uses/indications	constipation
Type of drug	POM, GSL
Presentation	tablets (green/brown), granules (brown), syrup (brown)
Dosage	1–2 tablets nocte, granules 5–10 mL nocte, syrup 10–20 mL nocte
Route of admin	oral
Contraindications	avoid abuse as it can cause atonic non-functioning colon and hypokalaemia
Side effects	abdominal cramps, local irritation
Interactions	no data available
Fetal risk	no reports of fetal or animal toxicity
Breastfeeding	standardized forms are considered safe

BP	GLYCEROL/GLYCERIN
Proprietary	non-proprietary, see BNF for details
Group	stimulant laxative – rectal stimulant only
Uses/indications	constipation
Type of drug	POM
Presentation	suppositories
Dosage	adult: 4 g = one suppository
Route of admin	p.r.
Contraindications	anal fissure, haemorrhoids
Side effects	local irritation
Interactions	N/A
Fetal risk	N/A
Breastfeeding	N/A

BP	LACTULOSE
Proprietary	Duphalac® (Solvay Healthcare Ltd), lactulose solution (Novartis Consumer Health), non-proprietary, see BNF for details
Group	osmotic laxative
Uses/indications	constipation
Type of drug	POM
Presentation	solution, white crystalline powder
Dosage	15 mL b.d. (50 % solution)
Route of admin	oral
Contraindications	galactosaemia, intestinal obstruction
Side effects	flatulence, abdominal cramps and discomfort
Interactions	no data available
Fetal risk	no reports of teratogenicity or hazard to the fetus
Breastfeeding	considered safe

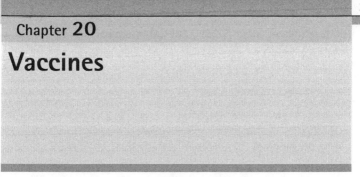

Chapter 20

Vaccines

A vaccine is a suspension of dead or disabled organisms which, when ingested or injected, prevents, lessens or treats infections or disease. The most commonly used vaccines in midwifery are rubella and varicella.

The student should be aware of:

- Detection of low levels of rubella antibodies in a client
- When it is appropriate to give vaccines in the postnatal period
- The sequlae of either vaccination or of disease
- The possible side effects of vaccination.

References

Briggs GG, Freeman RK, Yaffe SJ. Drugs in pregnancy and lactation: a reference guide to fetal and neonatal risk, 3rd edn. Baltimore: Williams & Wilkins, 1990

British Medical Association and the Royal Pharmaceutical Society of Great Britain. British national formulary. Number 43, March 2002. Bath: Bath Press, 2002

Hale T. Medications and mothers' milk, 9th edn. USA: Pharmasoft Publications, 2000

Hopkins SJ. Drugs and pharmacology for nurses, 13th edn. Edinburgh: Churchill Livingstone, 1999

SPC from the eMC, Erevax® SmithKline Beecham UK, updated on the eMC 26/07/02

For varicella see Chapter15 – immunoglobulins

BP	RUBELLA VACCINE
Proprietary	Erevax® (SmithKline Beecham UK)
Group	vaccine – live
Uses/indications	vaccination where there are low levels of rubella antibodies or none detected
Type of drug	POM
Presentation	ampoules, powder and solvent for reconstitution
Dosage	0.5 mL deep subcutaneous/IM
Route of admin	deep subcutaneous, IM
Contraindications	pregnancy or the intention to become pregnant within 1 month, febrile patients
Side effects	a mild form of the disease
Interactions	possible interference from passive antibodies, do not administer to subjects given human plasma or immunoglobulin in the previous 3 months
Pharmacodynamic properties	induces active immunization against rubella virus infection
Fetal risk	theoretical risk of teratogenicity and should therefore be avoided unless the need for vaccination outweighs the risk to the fetus
Breastfeeding	available data suggest that breastfeeding is safe

Chapter 21

Vitamins and Iron Preparations

Vitamins are factors in food necessary for growth and reproduction of living tissues. Some vitamins are fat soluble and others are water soluble.

Those of interest to the midwife are vitamins C, B_{12}, K and folic acid, and are usually present in the diet. Supplements of vitamins C and K are rare, but B_{12} and folic acid supplements are increasing.

Other elements present in food are minerals.

The student should be aware of:

- The importance of good nutrition in women of childbearing age
- What is considered malnutrition by the World Health Organization (WHO)
- The prevalence of malnutrition in local populations
- The sequelae to mother and fetus of malnutrition
- The foods which are part of a well balanced healthy diet.

IRON PREPARATIONS

Iron (Fe) is a metallic element and a constituent of the haemoglobin molecule that is necessary to carry oxygen around the body via the blood.

Involved in Fe absorption is vitamin C, and to a lesser extent folic acid. In theory, the haemoglobin (Hb) concentration in the blood should rise 2 g/100 ml or 20 g/L over 3–4 weeks of supplementation.

The student should be aware of:

- The WHO guidelines for diagnosis of anaemia
- The aetiology of and predisposing factors to anaemia
- The physiology and pathophysiology of anaemia in pregnancy
- The appropriateness and effectiveness of Fe preparations, both in anaemia and routinely in pregnancy
- The different kinds of anaemia and their prognosis
- The dietary sources of Fe, vitamin C and folic acid
- The sequelae of anaemia in the ante-, intra- and postnatal periods.

NB: Because of the risk of myocardial infarction Fe injections should be carried out under strict medical supervision. Defibrillation facilities and adrenaline (epinephrine) must be immediately available. It is also recommended that the course of oral Fe should be stopped 48 hours prior to the IM course.

Other Fe compounds

FEFOL Spansules® (Celltech Pharmaceuticals Ltd) – ferrous sulphate 150 mg and folic acid 500 μg – capsules (clear/green with brown, yellow and white pellets) – one capsule daily

Pregaday® (Celltech Pharmaceuticals Ltd) – ferrous fumarate (100 mg Fe) and folic acid (350 μg) tablets (brown) – one tablet daily.

References

Briggs GG, Freeman RK, Yaffe SJ. Drugs in pregnancy and lactation: a reference guide to fetal and neonatal risk, 3rd edn. Baltimore: Williams & Wilkins, 1990

British Medical Association and the Royal Pharmaceutical Society of Great Britain. British national formulary. Number 43, March 2002. Bath: Bath Press, 2002

Hale T. Medications and mothers' milk, 9th edn. USA: Pharmasoft Publications, 2000

Hopkins SJ. Drugs and pharmacology for nurses, 13th edn. Edinburgh: Churchill Livingstone, 1999

Little BB. Medication during pregnancy. In: James DK, Steer PJ, Weiner CP, Gonik B (eds) High risk pregnancy: management options, 2nd edn. London: WB Saunders, 1999; 617–638

Lloyd C, Lewis VM. Common medical disorders associated with pregnancy. In: Bennett VR, Brown LK (eds) Myles textbook for midwives, 13th edn. Edinburgh: Churchill Livingstone, 1999; 279–314

SPC from the eMC, Fefol Spansules®, Celltech Pharmaceuticals Ltd, updated from the eMC 25/02/02

SPC from the eMC, Pregaday®, Celltech Pharmaceuticals Ltd, updated from the eMC 25/01/02

SPC from the eMC, Jectofer®, AstraZeneca, updated from the eMC 12/04/02

Stockley IH (ed) Drug interactions. London: Pharmaceutical Press, 1999

BP	FERROUS SULPHATE
Proprietary	non-proprietary, see BNF for details
Group	Fe salts
Uses/indications	iron deficiency anaemia
Type of drug	POM
Presentation	tablets (white coated)
Dosage	one tablet 200 mg/day in prophylaxis or mild anaemia
	2–3 tablets 400–600 mg/daily in therapeutic doses
Route of admin	oral
Contraindications	diverticulitis, inflammatory bowel disease, anaemias other than iron deficiency, concurrent administration of parenteral iron
Side effects	nausea, gastric irritation, epigastric pain, diarrhoea or constipation, iron overload, darkening of the stools
Interactions	*antacids* – magnesium trisilicate reduces the absorption of Fe
	antibiotics – absorption of antibiotics can be reduced in the presence of Fe
Pharmacodynamic properties	iron aids haemoglobin regeneration and aids the oxidative processes in the tissues
Fetal risk	no data available
Breastfeeding	considered safe

BP	FE SORBITOL COMPOUND
Proprietary	Jectofer® (AstraZeneca)
Group	Fe salts
Uses/indications	failure of oral therapy, i. e. severe continuous blood loss, malabsorption
Type of drug	POM
Presentation	ampoules
Dosage	calculated according to client weight and iron deficiency – discontinue oral Fe 24 hrs prior to injection
	usually: 1.5 mg/kg body weight to a max. 100 mg/day
Route of admin	deep IM
Contraindications	liver and kidney disease (pyelonephritis), untreated urinary tract infection, early pregnancy, pre-existing cardiac anomalies
Side effects	pain at injection site, nausea, vomiting, dizziness, flushing, severe arrhythmias, theoretical risk of myocardial infarction, urine may turn black
Interactions	*chloramphenicol* – may delay response to iron treatment
Pharmacodynamic properties	absorption from the injection site is rapid and complete, and therefore rapidly increases Fe stores for utilization as required
Fetal risk	may cause teratogenicity or abortion in early pregnancy
Breastfeeding	no data

BP	FOLIC ACID
Proprietary	Preconceive® (Lane), non-proprietary, see BNF for details
Group	vitamins – B complex
Uses/indications	folate-deficient megaloblastic anaemia, preconception until 12 weeks' gestation prevention of neural tube defects
Type of drug	POM, GSL (doses must not exceed 500 μg/day)
Presentation	tablets, syrup
Dosage	400 μg daily preconception or for the first 12 weeks of gestation in anaemia: 5 mg/day for 4 months
Route of admin	oral
Contraindications	no data available
Side effects	no data available
Interactions	*antiepileptics* – folic acid is reduced by phenytoin or phenobarbital plasma concentration, therefore advice should be taken on supplementation.
Fetal risk	no data available on overdosage
Breastfeeding	considered safe

BP	VITAMIN B$_{12}$ HYDROXOCOBALAMIN
Proprietary	Cobalin-H®, Neo-Cytamen®, non-proprietary, see BNF for details
Group	vitamins – B complex
Uses/indications	**very rare in pregnancy**, pernicious anaemia, B$_{12}$ deficiency
Type of drug	POM
Presentation	ampoules
Dosage	1 mg repeat 5 times at 2–3-day intervals, maintenance dose 1 mg every 3 months
Route of admin	deep IM
Contraindications	diagnosis of deficiency should be fully established
Side effects	
Interactions	
Fetal risk	maternal B$_{12}$ deficiency results in poor fetal outcome – there are no reports of high maternal dosage at *term* and maternal or fetal complications
Breastfeeding	lack of B$_{12}$ in the maternal diet can cause neonatal anaemia. Dietary supplements are recommended where deficiency is diagnosed

Chapter 22

Anxiolytics and Hypnotics

These are used to lessen tension and excitement and to induce sleep. They may be prescribed for anxious patients or those unable to sleep in the antenatal period during hospitalization.

The student should be aware of:

- The effects tension has in exacerbating certain conditions
- The addictive qualities of such preparations.

References

Briggs GG, Freeman RK, Yaffe SJ. Drugs in pregnancy and lactation: a reference guide to fetal and neonatal risk, 3rd edn. Baltimore: Williams & Wilkins, 1990

British Medical Association and the Royal Pharmaceutical Society of Great Britain. British national formulary. Number 43, March 2002. Bath: Bath Press, 2002

Hale T. Medications and mothers' milk, 9th edn. USA: Pharmasoft Publications, 2000

Hopkins SJ. Drugs and pharmacology for nurses, 13th edn. Edinburgh: Churchill Livingstone, 1999

Little BB. Medication during pregnancy. In: James DK, Steer PJ, Weiner CP, Gonik B (eds) High risk pregnancy: management options, 2nd edn. London: WB Saunders, 1999; 617–638

SPC from the eMC, Temazepam 10 mg and 20 mg, Lagap Pharmaceuticals Ltd, updated on the eMC 07/08/97

Stockley IH (ed) Drug interactions. London: Pharmaceutical Press, 1999

BP	TEMAZEPAM
Proprietary	Temazepam (Lagap Pharmaceuticals Ltd), non-proprietary, see BNF for details
Group	hypnotic – benzodiazepine
Uses/indications	insomnia (short-term use)
Type of drug	POM (CD Schedule 3)
Presentation	tablets (white)
Dosage	10–20 mg nocte
Route of admin	oral
Contraindications	any history of drug/alcohol abuse, respiratory disease, myasthenia gravis, marked personality disorders, hypersensitivity to this or benzodiazepines, renal/hepatic disorder, sleep apnoea, muscle weakness
Side effects	drowsiness, lightheadedness, reduced alertness, confusion, fatigue, muscle weakness, numbed emotion, headache, ataxia, double vision
Interactions	*alcohol, analgesics, anaesthetics, antiepileptics, antihistamines, antihypertensives* – all enhance the sedatory effect *antihistamines* – concomitant administration with diphenhydramine can cause intrauterine or early neonatal death
Pharmacodynamic properties	a hypnotic/sedative/anxiolytic results in anxiolysis, muscle relaxation, CNS sedation, possibly acting on GABA receptors to potentiate GABA effects

table continues

Fetal risk	drowsiness, with large doses hypotonia, during last phase of pregnancy or during labour – depression of neonatal respiration, hypothermia and withdrawal symptoms
Breastfeeding	considered moderately safe but avoid repeated doses – can lead to lethargy and weight loss in the infant

Chapter **23**

Antifungals

These are drugs used to combat fungal infections. They can be ingested or applied topically, depending on the infection. The student should be aware of:

● Common antifungal infections in pregnancy
● The physiology and pathophysiology that allow these infections to flourish
● The appropriateness of the antifungal treatment prescribed.

References

Briggs GG, Freeman RK, Yaffe SJ. Drugs in pregnancy and lactation: a reference guide to fetal and neonatal risk, 3rd edn. Baltimore: Williams & Wilkins, 1990

British Medical Association and the Royal Pharmaceutical Society. British national formulary. Number 43, March 2002. Bath: Bath Press, 2002

Hale T. Medications and mothers' milk, 9th edn. USA: Pharmasoft Publications, 2000

Hopkins SJ. Drugs and pharmacology for nurses, 13th edn. Edinburgh: Churchill Livingstone, 1999

SPC from the eMC, Nystatin® oral suspension BP, Lagap Pharmaceuticals Ltd, accessed on the eMC 05/04/02

SPC from the eMC, Nystatin® pastilles, E.R. Squibb and Sons Ltd, updated on the eMC 20/08/01

SPC from the eMC, Nystatin® pessaries, E.R.Squibb and Sons Ltd, updated on the eMC 20/08/01

SPC from the eMC, Nystatin® vaginal cream, E.R.Squibb and Sons Ltd, updated on the eMC 24/08/01

SPC from the eMC, Canestan® pessary, Bayer PLC, updated on the eMC 13/12/01

SPC from the eMC, Candiden® pessary, Aventa Pharmaceuticals Ltd, updated on the eMC August 1999

BP	NYSTATIN
Proprietary	Nystan® (Lagap Pharmaceuticals Ltd, E.R. Squibb and Sons Ltd)
Group	antifungal
Uses/indications	candidiasis in the mouth, oesophagus or intestinal tract
Type of drug	POM
Presentation	oral suspension (yellow), tablets, pessaries, pastilles
Dosage	oral: 100 000 units q.d.s. for 7 days, i.e. one pastille or 1 mL of suspension vaginally: 1–2 pessaries for 12–14 nights intestinal infection: 5 mL q.d.s.
Route of admin	oral, per vaginam
Contraindications	
Side effects	nausea, vomiting, hypersensitivity
Interactions	no data available
Pharmacodynamic properties	antifungal which is not absorbed by the gastro-intestinal tract, skin or vagina, and which inhibits growth of microbes, mostly *Candida albicans*
Fetal risk	no reports of complications after administration in pregnancy
Breastfeeding	not secreted in breast milk

BP	CLOTRIMAZOLE
Proprietary	Canesten® (Bayer plc), Candiden® (Aventa Pharmaceuticals Ltd)
Group	antifungal
Uses/indications	candidiasis
Type of drug	POM, GSL
Presentation	cream (topical), pessaries
Dosage	see manufacturer's instructions
Route of admin	oral, per vaginam
Contraindications	hypersensitivity
Side effects	occasional local irritation
Interactions	*antifungals* – may reduce the efficacy of other drugs used in fungal disease, e.g. nystatin *contraceptives* – may affect latex condoms and diaphragms
Pharmacodynamic properties	broad-spectrum antifungal effective against proliferating fungi, e.g. yeast, mould, dermatophytes, as well as others. The anti-mycotic effect against the cell wall releases hydrogen peroxide and causes cell death
Fetal risk	use with caution as US studies show that when first-trimester vaginitis was treated with this preparation there was a small association with birth defects
Breastfeeding	considered safe as minimal absorption

Chapter 24

Miscellaneous

This chapter contains the drugs that are used in midwifery and which do not come under any previous title. They include some alternative medicines as well as pharmaceutical preparations. A recognized and registered practitioner in the alternative therapy should prescribe any such preparation, just as with conventional medicine one would seek the advice of a doctor or pharmacist prior to taking a medicine.

The student is urged to examine Rule 41, further expanded in the Midwives' Code of Practice (1998) and the more recent Guidelines for the Administration of Medicines (2000) for guidance when a client is using or wishes to use alternative therapies.

References

British Medical Association and the Royal Pharmaceutical Society of Great Britain. British national formulary. Number 43, March 2002. Bath: Bath Press, 2002

Hale T. Medications and mothers' milk, 9th edn. USA: Pharmasoft Publications, 2000

Hirvioja ML, Tuimala R, Vuori J. The treatment of intrahepatic cholestasis of pregnancy by dexamethasone. British Medical Journal 1992; 99:109–111

Hopkins SJ. Drugs and pharmacology for nurses, 13th edn. Edinburgh: Churchill Livingstone, 1999

Little BB. Medication during pregnancy. In: James DK, Steer PJ, Weiner CP, Gonik B (eds) High risk pregnancy: management options, 2nd edn. London: WB Saunders, 1999; 617–638

Lloyd C, Lewis VM. Common medical disorders associated with pregnancy. In: Bennett VR, Brown LK (eds) Myles textbook for midwives, 13th edn. Edinburgh: Churchill Livingstone, 1999; 279–314

RCOG. Antenatal corticosteroids to prevent respiratory distress syndrome. Clinical Greentop Guidelines no.7, December 1999

Reichen J. Intrahepatic cholestasis of pregnancy. 2002 *www.ikp.unibe.ch/lab2.html*

SPC from the eMC, Ursofalk®, Provalis Healthcare, updated on the eMC 22/08/01

SPC from the eMC, Urdox®, C.P. Pharmaceuticals Ltd, updated on the eMC 30/08/01

SPC from the eMC, Retrovir®, GlaxoSmithKline UK, updated on the eMC 23/05/02

SPC from the eMC, Zovirax® suspension, GlaxoSmithKline UK, updated on the eMC 17/08/01

SPC from the eMC, Zovirax®, 250 mg, 500 mg, GlaxoSmithKline UK, updated on the eMC 09/07/02

SPC from the eMC, Aciclovir®, Pharmacia, updated on the eMC 03/08/01

SPC from the eMC, Clomid®, Aventis Pharmaceuticals Ltd, updated on the eMC 23/08/01

SPC from the eMC, Eltroxin™ tablets, Goldshield Pharmaceuticals Ltd, accessed on the eMC 05/04/02

SPC from the eMC, Thyroxin BP 100 µg, 50 µg, 25 µg, Celltech Manufacturers Services Ltd, updated on the eMC 07/02/02

SPC from the eMC, Dexamethasone sodium phosphate BP, 8 mg/2 mL injection, Faulding Pharmaceuticals PLC, updated on the eMC 27/03/02

SPC from the eMC, Dexamethasone sodium phosphate BP, vials for injection, Organon Laboratories Ltd, updated on the eMC 17/04/02

SPC from the eMC, Betnesol®, Celltech Pharmaceuticals Ltd, updated on the eMC 09/07/01

Stockley IH (ed) Drug interactions. London: Pharmaceutical Press, 1999

Tiran D, Mack S (eds) Complementary therapies for pregnancy and childbirth. London: Baillière Tindall, 1995

http://www.medigraphic.com/pdfs/hepato/ah–2002pdf

www.bumc.bu.edu/www/busm/cme/modules/Jaundice_Preg/ihcp.htm#Treatment

BP	ZIDOVUDINE (AZT)
Proprietary	Retrovir® (GlaxoSmithKline UK)
Group	antiviral
Uses/indications	management of HIV, possibly in the prevention of materno-fetal HIV transmission
Type of drug	POM
Presentation	capsules (white/blue band and blue-white/dark blue band) syrup, powder for reconstitution, vials 200 mg in 20 mL solution (10 mg/ml)
Dosage	prevention of maternofetal transmission – over 14 weeks' gestation oral: 100 mg five times a day until labour
	labour and delivery: IVI 2 mg/kg over 1 hr then 1 mg/kg/hr until the cord is clamped. If LSCS planned then commence the regimen 4 hrs prior to delivery
Route of admin	oral, IV infusion
Contraindications	low haemoglobin or neutrophil counts, haematological toxicity: monitor blood levels
	vitamin B_{12} deficiency
Side effects	multiple, including gastrointestinal disturbances, headache, rash, fever, anaemia
Interactions	*analgesics* – methadone increases the plasma concentration of this drug

table continues

	antiepileptics – plasma phenytoin concentrations can increase or decrease; valproate – there is a potential for toxicity as plasma levels are increased
Pharmacodynamic properties	antiviral agent which acts as a virostatic by disrupting viral DNA to inhibit growth and reduce viral numbers
Fetal risk	use only if clearly indicated – possible maternal and fetal anaemia
Breastfeeding	not recommended

BP	ACICLOVIR (ACYCLOVIR)
Proprietary	Zovirax® (GlaxoWellcome), Aciclovir® (Pharmacia)
Group	anti-viral
Uses/indications	treatment of varicella zoster in pregnancy, herpes zoster, shingles and cold sores
Type of drug	POM
Presentation	powder for reconstitution, tablets
Dosage	IV infusion over 1 hr – 5 mg/kg t.d.s. oral: 800 mg × 5/day for 7 days
Route of admin	IV infusion, oral
Contraindications	renal impairment
Side effects	multiple including, rash, gastrointestinal disturbances, on IV infusion – local inflammation
Interactions	
Pharmacodynamic properties	a virostatic which interferes with the DNA reproduction function of the virus, reducing production and inhibiting its growth
Fetal risk	use only when the benefits outweigh the risks, as the number of exposures to the drug is too limited to assess the long-term prognosis
Breastfeeding	significant amount secreted into breast milk
	oral: 5-day course – considered safe
	IV: insufficient information to allow classification as safe

BP	THYROXINE (LEVOTHYROXINE)
Proprietary	Eltorxin™ (Goldshield Pharmaceuticals Ltd), Thyroxine BP (Celltech), non-proprietary, see BNF for details
Group	thyroid hormone
Uses/indications	hypothyroidism
Type of drug	POM
Presentation	tablets
Dosage	as indicated by laboratory monitoring and the physician
Route of admin	oral
Contraindications	thyrotoxicosis, hypersensitivity
Side effects	these usually occur with overdose – tachycardia, palpitations, muscle cramps and other indications of an increased metabolic rate
Interactions	*antidepressants* – tricyclics, amitriptyline – the antidepressant response is increased by the concurrent use of thyroxine *anticoagulants* – the effect of warfarin is enhanced *antiepileptics* – phenobarbitone and phenytoin accelerate the metabolism of thyroxine, phenytoin levels are increased by thyroxine *cimetidine* – reduces the absorption of thyroxine from the gut *cholestyramine* – the absorption of thyroxine is reduced *iron* – ferrous sulphate – reduced absorption of thyroxine

table continues

	hypoglycaemics – monitor insulin requirements because of increased metabolic rate *oral contraceptives* – may increase plasma levels of thyroxine
Pharmacodynamic properties	a naturally occurring hormone that contains iodine and is produced by the thyroid gland – required for growth, development and the nervous system. It also increases the basal metabolic rate and has stimulatory effects on heart and skeletal muscle, liver and kidneys
Fetal risk	monitor serum levels closely
Breastfeeding	maternal dosage may interfere with neonatal screening for hypothyroidism

BP	LOPERAMIDE
Proprietary	Imodium® (Janssen-Cilag)
Group	antidiarrhoeal
Uses/indications	acute/chronic diarrhoea
Type of drug	POM
Presentation	capsules, syrup
Dosage	adjusted according to response
Route of admin	oral
Contraindications	abdominal distension, acute ulcerative colitis
Side effects	abdominal cramps, urticaria
Interactions	no data available
Fetal risk	no reports found linking loperamide with either human or animal toxicity
Breastfeeding	one report in Australia recommends avoidance but otherwise no data are available, therefore it is considered safe

BP	DEXAMETHASONE
Proprietary	non-proprietary, see BNF for details
Group	glucocorticoid (steroid)
Uses/indications	to promote fetal lung surfactant production under 36 weeks' gestation and where labour is imminent/probable; can also ameliorate the effects of cholestasis of pregnancy
Type of drug	POM
Presentation	tablets, IM injection – ampoules
Dosage	RCOG guidelines: IM 6 mg 12 hrs apart for four doses (do not repeat after max. dose)
Route of admin	oral, IM
Contraindications	avoid in suspected chorioamnionitis, tuberculosis, porphyria
Side effects	rarely anaphylaxis, hypersensitivity, flushing, puerperal rash, fluid retention with repeated doses
Interactions	*analgesics* – increases the risk of gastrointestinal bleed with aspirin and other NSAIDs *antibiotics* – erythromycin may alter the metabolism of corticosteroids *anticoagulants* – alters the effects of anticoagulants, therefore monitor blood levels closely *antidiabetics* – antagonizes the hypoglycaemic effects

table continues

	antiepileptics – phenobarbitone, phenytoin and carbamazepine accelerate the metabolism of corticosteroids *antihypertensives* – antagonizes the antihypertensive effect
Pharmacodynamic properties	a glucocorticoid which has complex actions, one of which is to promote the production of lung surfactant. It is used to good effect when premature birth is anticipated and ameliorates the effects of cholestasis during pregnancy by reducing serum oestrogen levels. As premature delivery is an outcome of this condition it also contributes towards reducing neonatal mortality and morbidity
Fetal risk	overdose can affect the adrenal development of the fetus and neonate and may contribute to IUGR; however, the benefits vastly outweigh the risks of administration
Breastfeeding	no data available – but considered moderately safe if the benefits outweigh the risks

BP	BETAMETHASONE
Proprietary	Betnesol® (Celltech Pharmaceuticals Ltd)
Group	glucocorticoid (steroid)
Uses/indications	to promote fetal lung surfactant production under 36 weeks' gestation and where labour is imminent/probable
Type of drug	POM
Presentation	IM injection – ampoules
Dosage	RCOG guidelines: IM 12 mg 24 hrs apart, i.e. 24 mg in total (once only)
Route of admin	IM
Contraindications	avoid in suspected chorioamnionitis, tuberculosis, porphyria
Side effects	rarely anaphylaxis, hypersensitivity, flushing, puerperal rash, fluid retention with repeated doses
Interactions	*analgesics* – increases the risk of gastrointestinal bleed with aspirin and other NSAIDs *antibiotics* – erythromycin may alter the metabolism of corticosteroids *anticoagulants* – alters the effects of anticoagulants therefore monitor blood levels closely *antidiabetics* – antagonizes the hypoglycaemic effects *antiepileptics* – phenobarbitone, phenytoin and carbamazepine accelerate the metabolism of corticosteroids *antihypertensives* – antagonizes the antihypertensive effect

table continues

Pharmacodynamic properties	a glucocorticoid which has complex actions, one of which is to promote the production of lung surfactant. It is used to good effect when premature birth is anticipated
Fetal risk	fetal teratogenicity at organogenesis, overdosage can effect the adrenal development of the fetus and neonate and may contribute to IUGR; however, the benefits vastly outweigh the risks of administration
Breastfeeding	considered moderately safe as there are no controlled studies involving breastfeeding women and their infants

BP	CHLOMIPHENE CITRATE
Proprietary	Clomid® (Aventis Pharmaceuticals Ltd)
Group	anti-oestrogen
Uses/indications	anovulatory infertility
Type of drug	POM
Presentation	tablets
Dosage	50 mg/day for 5 days after the onset of menstruation; if no ovulation occurs after the first cycle then 100 mg for 5 days – use for a **maximum** of three cycles and under the supervision of a specialist centre
Route of admin	oral
Contraindications	**pregnancy**, hepatic disease, abnormal uterine bleeding, ovarian cysts except polycystic ovaries, CAUTION – with uterine fibroids
Side effects	menstrual symptoms, hot flushes, abdominal discomfort, withdraw if there are visual disturbances or ovarian hyperstimulation, hair loss, weight gain, rashes, dizziness, rarely convulsions
Interactions	
Pharmacodynamic properties	non-steroidal agent which stimulates ovulation in a high percentage of appropriately selected clients

table continues

| Fetal risk | fetal loss, ectopic pregnancy, risk of multiple pregnancy, multiple effects on fetal development, including neural tube defects and trisomies, reported – although not supported by data from population-based studies and still being investigated – therefore pregnancy should be excluded before the next course is commenced |
| Breastfeeding | considered hazardous and inhibits lactation |

NAME	HAMAMELIS VIRGINICA A.K.A. WITCH HAZEL
Proprietary	
Group	
Uses/indications	varicosities, perineal trauma, herpes lesions
Type of drug	herbal remedy
Presentation	liquid
Dosage	as directed by practitioner
Route of admin	topical
Contraindications	
Side effects	
Interactions	
Fetal risk	
Breastfeeding	

NAME	MARIGOLD, A.K.A. CALENDULA OFFICINALIS
Proprietary	
Group	
Uses/indications	perineal trauma, sore nipples, cystitis, thrush, herpes
Type of drug	herbal remedy
Presentation	ointment, infusion
Dosage	as directed by practitioner
Route of admin	oral or topical
Contraindications	
Side effects	
Interactions	
Fetal risk	
Breastfeeding	there is a possible risk of allergy which can cause anaphylaxis – therefore considered moderately safe as there are no studies showing increased adverse effects in breastfeeding infants

BP	PEPPERMINT WATER
Proprietary	
Group	
Uses/indications	to ease colic/flatulence and abdominal cramps
Type of drug	herbal remedy, also used in aromatherapy
Presentation	herbal tea: to treat anaemia and mood swings
	herbal suspension/infusion: as indicated above
	essential oil: to treat nausea and vomiting
Dosage	as directed by practitioner
Route of admin	oral, inhaled
Contraindications	
Side effects	
Interactions	
Fetal risk	
Breastfeeding	

NAME	ARNICA MONTANA A.K.A. LEOPARD'S BANE
Uses/indications	first-aid remedy in bruising and soreness, e.g. episiotomy or other perineal trauma
Type of drug	homeopathic remedy
Presentation	tablet or suspension
Dosage	as directed by homeopathic practitioner
Route of admin	oral
Contraindications	
Side effects	
Interactions	
Fetal risk	
Breastfeeding	

BP	URSODEOXYCHOLIC ACID (UDCA)
Proprietary	Ursofalk® (Provalis Healthcare), Urdox® (CP Pharmaceuticals), non-proprietary, see BNF for details
Group	acts on gallbladder
Uses/indications	dissolution of bile acids/gallstones, reduces itching and ameliorates liver enzymes, used in treatment of intrahepatic cholestasis of pregnancy (IHCP)
Type of drug	POM
Presentation	tablets, capsules, suspension
Dosage	Oral: 8–12 mg/kg/day (20–25 g/kg/day – effective and safe)
Route of admin	oral
Contraindications	pregnancy
Side effects	nausea, vomiting, diarrhoea, pruritus
Interactions	*antacids* – these bind to bile acids in the gut and have a detrimental effect on mode of action of UDCA *cholestyramine* – binds to bile acids in the gut and has a detrimental effect on mode of action of UDCA *oestrogens* – oral contraceptives – increased bile cholesterol is released, theoretically increasing the effective dose of UDCA
Pharmacodynamic properties	complex action, but when given orally UDCA dissolves bile acids in the biliary fluid and disperses them, reducing cholesterol and thus ameliorating the cholestasis

table continues

| Fetal risk | carcinogen in animal studies and manufacturers advise avoidance; however, the benefits may outweigh the risks in IHCP |
| Breastfeeding | manufacturer advises avoidance, but in the absence of controlled study data it is considered moderately safe when treating IHCP |

Chapter 25

Emergency Drugs

This chapter includes some of the drugs used in emergencies such as eclampsia and haemorrhage. Also included is a list of drugs used in cardiac arrest or during treatment of anaphylactic shock. These drugs are administered under the direct supervision of an expert, i.e. a consultant anaesthetist, and therefore the dosages are not included unless of course they are particularly relevant.

Each student should quickly become familiar with the local protocols and policies that cover such emergencies and seek adequate training in resuscitation techniques.

TREATMENT OF SEVERE HAEMORRHAGE

DRUGS USED IN THE TREATMENT OF CARDIAC ARREST

These drugs can be split into three sections: those used in primary treatment of cardiac arrest, those administered as secondary to stabilize the patient's condition, and those administered in the treatment of anaphylactic shock.

Primary – adrenaline (epinephrine)

Primary – lignocaine

Primary – atropine sulphate

Primary/secondary – calcium carbonate/calcium gluconate

Secondary – bicarbonate – usually sodium

Anaphylaxis – hydrocortisone
Anaphylaxis – chlorpheniramine.
Drugs used in neonatal resuscitation – narcan.

References

Baskett PJF. Resuscitation handbook, 2nd edn. London: Mosby-Wolfe, 1993

Briggs GG, Freeman RK, Yaffe SJ. Drugs in pregnancy and lactation: a reference guide to fetal and neonatal risk, 3rd edn. Baltimore: Williams & Wilkins, 1990

British Medical Association and the Royal Pharmaceutical Society of Great Britain. British national formulary. Number 43, March 2002. Bath: Bath Press, 2002

Hale T. Medications and mothers' milk, 9th edn. USA: Pharmasoft Publications, 2000

Hopkins SJ. Drugs and pharmacology for nurses, 13th edn. Edinburgh: Churchill Livingstone, 1999

Jevon P, Raby M. Resuscitation in pregnancy – a practical approach. Oxford: Books for Midwives, 2000

Little BB. Medication during pregnancy. In: James DK, Steer PJ, Weiner CP, Gonik B (eds) High risk pregnancy: management options, 2nd edn. London: WB Saunders, 1999; 617–638

SPC from the eMC, Diazemuls®, Dumex Ltd, updated on the eMC 02/08/01

SPC from the eMC, Heminevrin®, AstraZeneca, updated on the eMC 08/04/02

SPC from the eMC, magnesium sulphate injection 50%, Celltech Pharmaceuticals Ltd, updated on the eMC 13/08/02

SPC from the eMC, Haemabate®, Pharmacia, updated on the eMC 07/01/02

SPC from the eMC, atropine injection BP, Minijet, International Medication Systems (UK) Ltd, updated on the eMC 13/05/02

SPC from the eMC, lignocaine hydrochloride 1%, International Medication Systems (UK) Ltd, updated on the eMC 28/06/01

SPC from the eMC, Solu-Cortef®, Pharmacia, updated on the eMC 08/01/02

SPC from the eMC, Narcan neonatal®, 20 µg/mL, Bristol-Myers Squibb Pharmaceuticals Ltd, updated on the eMC 15/04/02

Stockley IH (ed) Drug interactions. London: Pharmaceutical Press, 1999

BP	ADRENALINE (EPINEPHRINE)
Proprietary	
Group	
Uses/indications	asystolic cardiac arrest in conjunction with calcium chloride and defibrillation. It increases cardiac output and the force of contractility by producing generalized vasoconstriction by acting on vascular smooth muscle. Can also be used in anaphylactic shock or severe allergic reactions
Type of drug	
Presentation	Minijet or ampoules
Dosage	0.5–1 mL of 1:10 000
Route of admin	IV
Contraindications	
Side effects	anxiety, tremor, increased heart rate, cold peripheries, increased blood pressure

BP	BICARBONATE – USUALLY SODIUM
Proprietary	
Group	
Uses/indications	used to combat metabolic acidosis after cardiac arrest. Should not be given until 20 minutes of cardiac arrest has elapsed

BP	CALCIUM CARBONATE/CALCIUM GLUCONATE
Proprietary	
Group	
Uses/indications	the calcium ions help to increase myocardial contractility when adrenaline has failed. Can be used in conjunction with adrenaline and defibrillation

BP	HYDROCORTISONE
Proprietary	Solu-Cortef® (Pharmacia)
Group	corticosteroids
Uses/indications	in anaphylaxis, in suppression of the inflammatory response
Type of drug	
Presentation	ampoules
Dosage	
Route of admin	IM, IV
Contraindications	
Side effects	
Interactions	
Pharmacodynamic properties	a glucocorticosteroid that suppresses the inflammatory response during anaphylaxis
Fetal risk	
Breastfeeding	

BP	CHLORPHENIRAMINE
Proprietary	Piriton® (Stafford-Miller Ltd)
Group	antihistamine – see Chapter 12
Uses/indications	in anaphylaxis, in suppression of severe inflammatory response
Type of drug	
Presentation	see Chapter 12
Dosage	continuous IV infusion over 24 hrs – 10–20 mg as an adjunct to epinephrine (adrenaline)

BP	PHENYTOIN
Proprietary	Epanutin® (Parke Davis)
Group	anti-epileptic
Uses/indications	epilepsy, eclampsia
Type of drug	POM
Presentation	capsules, tablets, suspension
Dosage	see local protocols
Route of admin	oral, IV infusion or injection, p.r.
Contraindications	see Chapter 6
Side effects	see Chapter 6
Interactions	see Chapter 6
Pharmacodynamic properties	see Chapter 6
Fetal risk	see Chapter 6
Breastfeeding	see Chapter 6

DRUGS USED IN THE TREATMENT OF SEVERE PRE-ECLAMPSIA AND ECLAMPSIA

BP	MAGNESIUM SULPHATE (SEE BNF FOR DETAILS)
Proprietary	
Group	anticonvulsant – muscle relaxant
Uses/indications	in pre-eclampsia and eclampsia
Type of drug	POM
Presentation	ampoules
Dosage	according to local protocol, typically: IV 4 g over 5–10 minutes, then by IVI 1 g every hour for 24 hrs
	recurrent seizures: IV bolus 2 g monitor heart rate, BP, respiration, urinary output and reflexes; see BNF for details
Route of admin	IV infusion
Contraindications	
Side effects	OVERDOSE – loss of patellar reflexes, weakness, nausea, sensation of warmth, flushing, drowsiness, slurred speech, double vision
Interactions	*caution with aminoglycoside antibiotics* within the first 24–48 hrs of birth
	because of the risk of respiratory depression do not combine *barbiturates, opioids or hypnotics*

table continues

Pharmacodynamic properties	magnesium is involved in neurochemical transmission and muscular excitability and acts as a depressant on the CNS, and peripherally causes vasodilation. IV administration has an immediate effect and lasts for approximately 30 minutes
Fetal risk	fetal heart rate should be monitored continuously, neurological depression of the neonate includes respiratory depression, muscle weakness and loss of reflexes
Breastfeeding	secreted but considered safe
Antagonist	calcium gluconate

NB: According to the BNF and SPC ECG monitoring is required during administration as BP and observation for signs of overdose

BP	CHLOARIMETHIAZOLE
Proprietary	Heminevrin® (AstraZeneca)
Group	hypnotic, anxiolytic
Uses/indications	eclampsia
Type of drug	POM
Presentation	capsules, syrup, IV infusion
Dosage	see local protocol
Route of admin	IV (oral)
Contraindications	pulmonary insufficiency
Side effects	
Interactions	*alcohol* – enhances the sedative effect *anaesthesia* – enhances the sedative effect *analgesics* – opioids enhance the sedative effect *antihistamines* – enhance the sedative effect *antihypertensives* – enhance the hypotensive effect
Pharmacodynamic properties	a sedative muscle relaxant with anticonvulsant properties. When given alone it has little effect on respiration
Fetal risk	can depress neonatal respiration
Breastfeeding	amount secreted too small to be harmful

BP	NALOXONE
Proprietary	Narcan® (Bristol-Myers Squibb)
Group	antagonist of central and respiratory depression
Uses/indications	reversal of the effects of opioid analgesia in neonates
Type of drug	POM
Presentation	ampoules
Dosage	200 μg single dose at birth. This dose is for a term infant only and a preterm infant requires a smaller dose – this should be agreed with the paediatrician in attendance at delivery
Route of admin	IM, subcutaneous
Contraindications	
Side effects	
Interactions	
Pharmacodynamic properties	an opioid antagonist that is devoid of the morphine-like properties of other antagonists. It acts within 2 minutes of IV administration but takes longer with IM or s.c. administration, although its effects via these routes last longer
Fetal risk	
Breastfeeding	

BP	DIAZEPAM
Proprietary	Diazemuls® (Dumex Ltd)
Group	benzodiazepine – sedative, hypnotic, muscle relaxant
Uses/indications	short-term anxiety/insomnia, status epilepticus, eclampsia
Type of drug	POM
Presentation	tablets, solution, emulsion, suppositories
Dosage	oral: anxiety 2 mg t.d.s. increasing to 5–30 mg daily, else refer to protocol
	suppositories: rectal solution 5–15 mg
	slow IV: 5–10 mg repeated not less than 4-hrly
Route of admin	oral, IM, IV, p.r.
Contraindications	history of drug or alcohol dependence, existing respiratory depression, mental illness including psychosis and phobia, **pregnancy and breastfeeding**
Side effects	drowsiness, lightheadedness, confusion, **dependence**, after IV injection there may be a fall in blood pressure and severe respiratory depression
Interactions	*alcohol* – enhances sedative effect *anaesthesia* – enhances sedative effect *antiepileptics* – reported to both increase and decrease plasma phenytoin concentration, *antihistamines* – enhanced sedative effect *antihypertensives* – enhanced hypotensive effect

table continues

Pharmacodynamic properties	a potent anxiolytic, anticonvulsant and central muscle relaxant that mediates its effects via the limbic system and the postsynaptic spinal reflexes
Fetal risk	teratogen in the first and second trimesters, prolonged use in the third trimester may cause neonatal respiratory depression, drowsiness, hypotonia and withdrawal
Breastfeeding	moderately safe in the short term but avoid repeated doses and observe the infant for lethargy and weight loss. With long-term use see Fetal risk

BP	SODIUM CITRATE
Proprietary	
Group	antacid
Uses/indications	to reduce the acidity of gastric contents
Type of drug	POM
Presentation	solution
Dosage	30 ml immediately prior to the induction of anaesthesia
Route of admin	oral

BP	CIMETIDINE
Proprietary	see Chapter 1
Group	antacid
Uses/indications	labour where there is a high probability of LSCS, prior to emergency LSCS
Type of drug	POM
Presentation	tablets (green), pre-prepared ampoules for IV administration
Dosage	oral: 400 mg 6–8-hrly IV injection: slowly over 12 minutes – 200 mg
Route of admin	oral, IV
Contraindications	see Chapter 1
Side effects	see Chapter 1
Interactions	see Chapter 1
Pharmacodynamic properties	see Chapter 1
Fetal risk	see Chapter 1
Breastfeeding	see Chapter 1

BP	CARBOPROST
Proprietary	Haemabate® (Pharmacia)
Group	prostaglandin
Uses/indications	postpartum haemorrhage unresponsive to ergometrine or syntocinon
Type of drug	POM
Presentation	ampoules – 250 µg/mL
Dosage	250 µg repeated as required at 90-minute intervals – in severe loss not less than 15 minutes
	total dose is 2 mg maximum, i.e. eight doses
Route of admin	deep IM
Contraindications	untraced pelvic infection, cardiac, pulmonary, hepatic or renal disease, caution in asthma, hypertension or hypotension, anaemia, jaundice, diabetes, epilepsy, uterine scarring – an excessive amount of carboprost can cause uterine rupture
Side effects	multiple, including nausea, vomiting, hyperthermia, flushing, bronchospasm, possible need for oxygen therapy as there may be a reduction in maternal oxygen saturations
Interactions	

table continues

Pharmacodynamic properties	a synthetic prostaglandin stimulant with a longer action than dinoprost. It stimulates the uterus to contract as it would post delivery, and results in haemostasis at the site of placentation and prevents further blood loss, but the exact mechanism of action is unknown. It will also affect other receptors in other organs and systems, i.e. the gastrointestinal tract, the CNS, the urinary system and metabolic processing
Fetal risk	not applicable
Breastfeeding	not applicable

BP	LIGNOCAINE
Proprietary	Lignocaine hydrochloride 1% and 2% (IMS)
Group	
Uses/indications	after acute myocardial infarction it suppresses ventricular arrhythmias and reduces the potential for fibrillation and its recurrence. It decreases myocardial contractility and arterial blood pressure, and can be used where there is persistent ventricular fibrillation or ventricular tachycardia
Presentation	Minijet, ampoules
Dosage	slowly over 2 minutes – 1 mg/kg – bolus 0.5 mg/kg after 5–10 minutes
Route of admin	IV

BP	ATROPINE SULPHATE
Proprietary	Atropine injection BP Minijet (IMS)
Group	
Uses/indications	increases the heart rate by blocking the action of the vagus nerve on the sinus node. It is used in sinus bradycardia, especially where there is a drop in blood pressure following myocardial infarction. It can also be used in asystolic cardiac arrest which is unresponsive to DC shock
Type of drug	
Presentation	Minijet – injection
Dosage	1–3 mg

Drug Calculations

$$\frac{\text{required strength}}{\text{available strength}} \times \frac{\text{quantity preparation}}{\text{is supplied in}}$$

or

$$\frac{\text{what you want}}{\text{what you've got}} \times \text{IT (the preparation)}$$

e.g. ampicillin elixir 125 mg/5 mL the prescription says 100 mg, therefore:

$$\frac{100}{125} \times 5 = 4 \text{ mL}$$

Benzyl penicillin 600 mg/5 mL the prescription says 200 mg, therefore:

$$\frac{200}{600} \times 5 = 1.66 \text{ mL}$$

For rates of infusion

$$\text{Drops/min} = \frac{\text{drops/mL of giving set} \times \text{volume of infusion (mL)}}{\text{number of hrs to run} \times 60}$$

If the infusion is to run over minutes then divide by the number of minutes to run.

$$\text{ml/hr} = \frac{\text{total volume to be infused} \times \text{dose} \times 60}{\text{total amount of drug}}$$

$$\text{drops/min} = \frac{\text{total volume to be infused (mL)} \times \text{dose}}{\text{total amount of drug} \times \text{drip rate}}$$
$$\text{of giving set}$$

Reference

Laplain R, Agar H. Drug calculations for nurses. A step by step approach. London: Arnold, 995; 129–189

Index

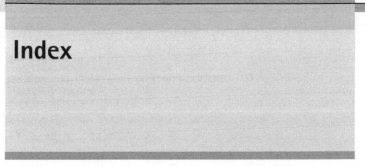

Headings in italics indicate proprietary names, or micro-organism

UNIVERSITIES AT MEDWAY LIBRARY